Dyslipidaemia in Cl:

T0231889

Dyslipidaemia in Clinical Practice
Second Edition

Gilbert Thompson MD FRCP
Emeritus Professor of Clinical Lipidology
Division of Investigative Science, Imperial College
Hammersmith Hospital
London
UK

Jonathan Morrell MB BChir FRCGP DCH DRCOG
General Practitioner
Beaconsfield Road Surgery
Hastings
East Sussex
UK

Peter Wilson MD
Professor of Medicine
Dept of Endocrinology, Diabetes, and Medical Genetics
Medical University of South Carolina
Charlston, SC
USA

Foreword by
Antonio M. Gotto, Jr MD DPhil

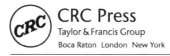

CRC Press
Taylor & Francis Group
Boca Raton London New York

CRC Press is an imprint of the
Taylor & Francis Group, an **informa** business

CRC Press
Taylor & Francis Group
6000 Broken Sound Parkway NW, Suite 300
Boca Raton, FL 33487-2742

© 2006 by Taylor & Francis Group, LLC
CRC Press is an imprint of Taylor & Francis Group, an Informa business

No claim to original U.S. Government works

This book contains information obtained from authentic and highly regarded sources. Reasonable efforts have been made to publish reliable data and information, but the author and publisher
cannot assume responsibility for the validity of all materials or the consequences of their use. The
authors and publishers have attempted to trace the copyright holders of all material reproduced in
this publication and apologize to copyright holders if permission to publish in this form has not
been obtained. If any copyright material has not been acknowledged please write and let us know so
we may rectify in any future reprint.

Except as permitted under U.S. Copyright Law, no part of this book may be reprinted, reproduced,
transmitted, or utilized in any form by any electronic, mechanical, or other means, now known or
hereafter invented, including photocopying, microfilming, and recording, or in any information
storage or retrieval system, without written permission from the publishers.

For permission to photocopy or use material electronically from this work, please access www.
copyright.com (http://www.copyright.com/) or contact the Copyright Clearance Center, Inc.
(CCC), 222 Rosewood Drive, Danvers, MA 01923, 978-750-8400. CCC is a not-for-profit organization that provides licenses and registration for a variety of users. For organizations that have been
granted a photocopy license by the CCC, a separate system of payment has been arranged.

Trademark Notice: Product or corporate names may be trademarks or registered trademarks, and
are used only for identification and explanation without intent to infringe.

Visit the Taylor & Francis Web site at
http://www.taylorandfrancis.com

and the CRC Press Web site at
http://www.crcpress.com

Contents

Foreword to second edition

As noted in the Foreword to the first edition of this book, by now, both cardiologists and primary care physicians have accepted dyslipidaemia as a major, treatable cause of atherosclerotic cardiovascular disease. In 2004, an article on the management of dyslipidaemia was one of the top ten most downloaded articles from the online version of *Heart*, a major cardiology journal, illustrating the relevance and timeliness of this topic. Rapid advances in knowledge in this field, especially insights gained from recent clinical trials, have helped shape new European and British guidelines on the prevention of cardiovascular disease and a revision of the US National Cholesterol Education Program's Adult Treatment Panel (ATP) III guidelines emphasizes the importance of radically reducing low-density lipoprotein (LDL) cholesterol in individuals who have or who are at very high risk for coronary heart disease. The ATP III argues that patients with type II diabetes who have not had a heart attack should receive as aggressive an approach as those with a history of heart disease. Furthermore, patients with the metabolic syndrome, a cluster of risk factors that enhances the risk for cardiovascular disease, require clinical attention, as well. These refinements, among others, in our understanding of cardiovascular risk and its treatment thus make necessary this second edition of *Dyslipidaemia in Clinical Practice*.

The ability to achieve the lower target levels of LDL cholesterol in the highest risk patients, as advocated in the revised version of ATP III, reflects changes in the pharmacologic armamentarium, such as newer, more potent statins and the cholesterol absorption blocker ezetimibe, which acts in an additive manner when given with a statin. These therapeutic advances together with advances in the epidemiology and genetics of dyslipidaemia, the increasing use of nutritional supplements, and improvements in the non-invasive detection of sub-clinical vascular disease are all dealt with in this second edition, with substantial revision by its authors, who comprise a lipidologist, a primary care physician, and an epidemiologist. Calling on their diverse expertises ensures that an appropriate balance is achieved between communicating basic knowledge of the underlying causes of dyslipidaemia and the practicalities of screening for and treating the disorder in a busy clinical setting.

The study of dyslipidaemia and its clinical cardiovascular implications is complex and fraught with challenges and controversies. Readers are in good hands under the guidance of Doctors Thompson, Morrell, and Wilson, as they survey this constantly evolving field. In its scope and content, *Dyslipidaemia in Clinical Practice* (2nd edition) is a valuable resource to clinicians who treat lipid disorders.

Antonio M. Gotto, Jr MD DPhil
Weill Medical College of Cornell University
New York, NY

Preface

The management of dyslipidaemia has become an important topic for health professionals working not only in primary care, but also in hospital, where the impact of dyslipidaemia is experienced across a wide range of medical and surgical specialities. Although now routine, it is important to remember that only in the last decade has dealing with dyslipidaemia become an established part of clinical practice. The acquisition and application of new knowledge has been rapid and this second edition of *Dyslipidaemia in Clinical Practice* has been extensively rewritten to bring the reader up to date with both new information and current issues for patient care.

What has not changed is the worldwide burden of cardiovascular disease and the need to tackle dyslipidaemia. The problem is as relevant in the developed societies of Europe and North America as it is in the developing world, where unhealthy lifestyle habits are burgeoning. Across the emergent spectrum of atherosclerotic vascular disease (coronary heart disease, cerebrovascular disease and peripheral arterial disease) dyslipidaemia remains of central importance both in terms of causation and therapeutic modification to reduce disability and death from these sequelae.

Since publication of the first edition, the expanding evidence base has confirmed the benefit of modifying dyslipidaemia for a spectrum of individuals with a wider range of cardiovascular risk. For individuals at high cardiovascular risk, lowering low-density lipoprotein (LDL) cholesterol by 1 mmol/L can be expected to reduce cardiovascular events by 20%, irrespective of age, sex or baseline values. For individuals at very high risk, more radical reduction of LDL cholesterol produces further benefits, and international guidelines advocate lower target levels to reflect this new evidence. The greatest benefits in cardiovascular event reduction seem to result from the greatest absolute LDL cholesterol reductions and new therapies have emerged capable of achieving the low levels required. The risk reductions seen in hypercholesterolaemic patients in clinical trials are remarkably consistent and have also been seen in patients with type 2 diabetes mellitus and hypertension. Even patients with lower degrees of cardiovascular risk benefit from lipid modification, albeit that the absolute benefits may be less. The threshold level of cardiovascular risk for lipid modification is defined not only by clinical effectiveness and acceptability, but also affordability, the latter especially since simvastatin became available as a generic drug in many countries.

In terms of effective health care delivery, most of the burden for lowering cardiovascular risk falls on individuals working in primary care. Primary care is well placed to tackle the enormity of the task and its holistic, multidisciplinary nature is well suited to multiple risk factor management and the establishment of the sort of therapeutic alliances that are so important for long-term treatment concordance. The introduction of performance related incentives for the management of chronic disease in the UK has resulted in spectacular improvements in the treatment of dyslipidaemia. For example, in patients with coronary heart disease, the target cholesterol of <5.0 mmol/L was reached in 71% of patients by April 2005. Lower drug acquisition costs and thresholds for intervention, however, raise concerns about increasing workloads and these remain real issues for a hard-pressed, resource-constrained and demand-led service.

Like hypertension and diabetes mellitus, dyslipidaemia is a complex subject. Dyslipidaemia means more than just elevated cholesterol, and other abnormalities of the lipoprotein profile and lipid metabolism are relevant. In particular, the pattern of low high density lipoprotein (HDL) cholesterol with raised triglycerides, so often seen in people with metabolic syndrome or diabetes mellitus, is under scrutiny as the incidence of those conditions increases to epidemic proportions. The current dominance of LDL cholesterol-lowering therapy is likely to lessen in the future with the emergence of new data and new approaches to raising HDL cholesterol and lowering triglyceride concentrations. Combination lipid-lowering drug strategies seem likely to proliferate, much as multiple drug therapy is now the norm in hypertension.

The complexity of the subject, the rapid development of new strategies and guidelines, the continuing influence of genetic and environmental factors and the emergence of a series of management issues relating to the treatment of dyslipidaemia mean that health professionals have a continuing need for clinical information on this topic. The aims of this book, therefore, remain the same as the first edition, namely to provide the reader with an up-to-date review of the pathophysiology and relevance of dyslipidaemia, the identification and assessment of affected individuals and a comprehensive account of their management, aimed at reducing death and disability from cardiovascular disease.

Acknowledgements

We thank Alan Burgess for suggesting we write a second edition of our book and Oliver Walter for encouraging and helping us to produce it. We are indebted, yet again, to Elizabeth Manson for her expert secretarial assistance with the manuscript. We are also very grateful to Tony Gotto for writing the Foreword, despite his numerous responsibilities and heavy workload.

Executive summary

PATHOPHYSIOLOGY OF PLASMA LIPIDS

Chapter 1 describes plasma lipids and the disorders which affect them. The main physiological systems involved in the absorption, metabolism, and storage of cholesterol and triglyceride are the small intestine, liver, adipose tissue and peripheral cells. These lipids are transported together with phospholipids within plasma by lipoproteins, which vary in size, composition and function. Dietary cholesterol and triglycerides are carried by chylomicrons and endogenously synthesized triglycerides by very low density lipoprotein. Cholesterol is transported out to the periphery by low density lipoprotein (LDL) and returned thence to the liver by high density lipoprotein (HDL). Most of the receptors, ligands and enzymes involved in lipoprotein metabolism have now been identified, often as a result of studying inborn errors. Other factors which influence prevailing levels of lipids in plasma include age, hormonal changes, diet, exercise and intercurrent illnesses.

Abnormal levels of plasma lipids are termed dyslipidaemia, which includes potentially pathological decreases in HDL as well as increases in any of the lipoprotein classes. Hyperlipidaemia and hypolipidaemia can each be primary, genetically-determined disorders or secondary, acquired disorders. Primary hyperlipidaemias are subdivided into hypercholesterolaemia, hypertriglyceridaemia or mixed hyperlipidaemia, where both cholesterol and triglycerides are elevated.

Genetically-determined causes of primary hypercholesterolaemia are familial hypercholesterolaemia, commonly due to mutations of the LDL receptor; familial defective apoB-100, due to point mutations of apoB-100; cholesterol ester storage disease, due to mutations of lysosomal cholesterol ester hydrolase; phytosterolaemia, due to mutations of ATP-binding cassette (ABC) transporters G5 and G8; and cerebrotendinous xanthomatosis, due to mutations of sterol 27α-hydrolase. Genetically-determined primary hypertriglyceridaemias include familial lipoprotein lipase deficiency and familial apoC-II deficiency, due to mutations of the corresponding genes, and familial hypertriglyceridaemia, the cause of which has yet to be discovered. Genetically-determined primary mixed hyperlipidaemias are type III hyperlipoproteinaemia, due to mutations of apoE; familial hepatic lipase deficiency, due to mutations of that enzyme; and familial combined hyperlipidaemia, the genetic basis of which is currently under intense scrutiny by several research groups.

Secondary hyperlipidaemia can be due to hormonal influences such as pregnancy, exogenous sex hormones or hypothyroidism; to metabolic disorders such as diabetes and obesity; to renal dysfunction or obstructive liver disease; to beverages, such as alcohol and coffee; and to iatrogenic causes, such as cyclosporin, amiodarone, retinoids and antiretroviral drugs.

Primary hypolipoproteinaemia (hypolipidaemia) is always of genetic origin and includes aβlipoproteinaemia, due to recessively inherited mutations of microsomal triglyceride transport protein (MTP); familial hypoβlipoproteinaemia, due to dominantly inherited mutations of the apoB gene leading to a truncated protein; Tangier disease, due to homozygosity for mutations of ABCA1; and familial hypoalphalipoproteinaemia, which can be due to heterozygous inheritance of mutations of either the ABCA1 or LCAT genes, or occasionally to mutations of apoA-1.

Finally, secondary hypolipoproteinaemia can be spontaneous, due to intestinal malabsorption, or surgically induced, as in partial ileal bypass.

DYSLIPIDAEMIA AS A RISK FACTOR FOR CARDIOVASCULAR DISEASE

Chapter 2 summarizes the various lines of epidemiological evidence which support the role of dyslipidaemia as a major risk factor for cardiovascular disease. Geographical differences in the severity of atherosclerosis and mortality from cardiovascular disease were shown to be associated with the high intakes of dietary saturated fat and cholesterol prevalent in Western countries in the 1960s and were accompanied by increased levels of plasma cholesterol, whereas the opposite applied to countries like Japan. The importance of diet was confirmed by studies of migrants from Japan to the USA, and several prospective studies of cardiovascular disease (CVD) incidence established that this reflected the influence of diet on plasma cholesterol. Further studies differentiated between the roles of LDL and HDL cholesterol, raised levels of the former increasing the risk of CVD, whereas raised levels of HDL had a protective effect. The latter phenomenon explained the lower mortality of premenopausal women, who have higher levels of HDL cholesterol than men.

In the past the risks associated with dyslipidaemia were usually expressed in relative terms but the tendency now is to define risk in absolute terms. Relative risk tends to be favoured by clinicians, who deal with individuals, whereas absolute risk is preferred by epidemiologists and health economists, who deal with populations.

The links between diet, plasma cholesterol and atherosclerosis are further supported by changing trends in coronary heart disease (CHD) mortality in countries such as the USA and Australia, where public health measures have been vigorously implemented, whereas the opposite is occurring in Eastern Europe and developing countries with recently acquired Westernized lifestyles.

DIETARY AND LIFESTYLE FACTORS IN DYSLIPIDAEMIA

Chapter 3 considers in greater detail the relationship between dyslipidaemia, diet and other lifestyle habits. The relationship between changes in the saturated and/or polyunsaturated fat content of the diet and changes in plasma cholesterol, mainly reflecting LDL cholesterol, can be estimated on the basis of mathematical formulae. Saturated fat increases LDL cholesterol whereas polyunsaturated fat has an opposite but weaker effect. Decreases in plasma cholesterol in countries such as the USA and Finland have been shown to be largely due to favourable changes in national diets, whereas the opposite is now occurring in Japan.

The well-established role of a raised level of LDL as a risk factor for CVD should not be allowed to overshadow the equal importance of a low level of HDL cholesterol. Factors which contribute to the latter are obesity, physical inactivity and diabetes, whereas moderate consumption of alcohol and exercise have the opposite effect. Intervention trials have demonstrated that dietary change results in a decrease in plasma cholesterol and that every 1% decrease is accompanied by a 2% decrease in the incidence of CHD. Emphatic confirmation of this relationship has subsequently come from the statin trials.

SCREENING FOR DYSLIPIDAEMIA

Chapter 4 discusses the question of how and whom to screen for dyslipidaemia. The establishment of a screening programme in a primary care setting requires a staged approach, first priority being given to screening those with established CHD, cerebrovascular disease, peripheral vascular disease or diabetes mellitus. The next priority should be to screen all those whose risk of cardiovascular risk may be high by virtue of either their risk factor profile or concomitant disease such as renal impairment or HIV infection. Other high-risk groups include those with a family history of premature CVD and relatives of patients with familial hypercholesterolaemia. Subsequently, opportunistic screening should be extended to all adults in the practice, 70% of whom visit their primary health care physician at least once a year. Screening for dyslipidaemia is not done in isolation, and other risk factors such as hypertension and smoking should also be sought. Recommendations for estimation of overall risk of CVD and the management of various degrees of dyslipidaemia in Britain are laid out in national guidelines.

CLINICAL ASSESSMENT OF DYSLIPIDAEMIA

Chapter 5 discusses the management of an individual found to be dyslipidaemic. This starts with a history and examination, including a search for corneal arcus and xanthomas. Laboratory investigations should include a full lipid profile, after an overnight fast, with calculation of LDL cholesterol and the total:HDL cholesterol ratio. Other investigations should include measurement of blood pressure, fasting glucose and a resting ECG. Quantification of both absolute and relative risk of future CHD should be undertaken with the aid of Framingham-based charts or computer programs. Risk factors for which there are insufficient data to merit inclusion in such estimates but which can be used in a qualitative manner include family history of premature CHD, Lp(a) and fibrinogen.

Because of the limitations of risk assessment it is worth seeking evidence of preclinical atherosclerosis using whatever non-invasive indices of vascular disease are available locally. These include carotid ultrasound to measure carotid intimal-medial thickness, computed tomography to measure coronary calcification and brachial ultrasound to measure flow-mediated arterial dilatation. Evidence of preclinical disease indicates the need for lipid-regulating drug therapy in an asymptomatic individual with diet-resistant dyslipidaemia.

GUIDELINES FOR THE MANAGEMENT OF DYSLIPIDAEMIA

Chapter 6 describes the various guidelines which have been issued over the years on the management of dyslipidaemia in the context of the primary and secondary prevention of CHD. Earlier guidelines were hampered by lack of proof that LDL-lowering therapy reduced total mortality, but the results of the statin trials have now proved conclusively that it does.

Recent guidelines have been issued by the Joint British Societies and Joint European Societies and the current US National Cholesterol Education Program (NCEP) Adult Treatment Panel (ATP) III guidelines were recently revised. All stress that secondary prevention should take precedence over primary prevention and that the latter should be focused on those found to have a high overall risk of CHD. The revised ATP III guidelines advocate even lower target levels of LDL cholesterol, often necessitating radical therapy, in those with CHD or at high risk.

PHARMACOLOGICAL MANAGEMENT OF DYSLIPIDAEMIA

Chapter 7 describes the rationale for lipid-regulating drug therapy and the evidence from angiographic and clinical outcome trials on which this is based. The three main classes of drug in use at the present time are the fibrates, bile acid sequestrants and HMG CoA reductase inhibitors or statins. The choice of which to use will depend upon the type of dyslipidaemia to be treated, fibrates being the most effective means of lowering triglycerides and raising HDL cholesterol, and statins the most effective in lowering LDL cholesterol. Bile acid sequestrants are usually reserved for patients with a raised LDL in whom safety is a paramount concern, such as children and fertile females. All three classes of drug have a substantial body of evidence to support their efficacy and safety, especially the statins. The latter have revolutionized the treatment and prevention of CHD during the past five years and are being increasingly used as patents expire and cheaper, generic products become available.

Other compounds which merit a mention are nicotinic acid, use of which is restricted by its side-effects, and ω-3 fatty acids. Patients with severe dyslipidaemia may require combination drug therapy, which usually involves concomitant administration of one of the statins with either a bile acid sequestrant or ezetimibe, if hypercholesterolaemia is the main concern, or with a fibrate in patients with mixed dyslipidaemia who fail to respond to statin monotherapy. Severe hypertriglyceridaemia may necessitate the combination of a fibrate and nicotinic acid or large doses of ω-3 fatty acids.

Recent developments include the introduction of rosuvastatin, which appears to be even more effective in lowering LDL cholesterol than atorvastatin, and the cholesterol absorption inhibitor, ezetimibe, which is proving to be a valuable adjunct to statins in patients who respond poorly to the latter or cannot tolerate a high dose. Although the current emphasis is on lowering LDL cholesterol, it is likely that in the not too distant future the emphasis will shift to compounds aimed at raising HDL cholesterol. Foremost among these is the cholesterol ester transfer protein (CETP) inhibitor torcetrapib, currently undergoing clinical trials. Such developments will enable physicians to treat dyslipidaemia with ever-increasing efficiency and thereby reduce still further the burden of CVD in clinical practice.

MANAGEMENT ISSUES IN PRIMARY CARE

Chapter 8 focuses on the logistics of managing dyslipidaemia in a primary care setting and stresses that this should be an holistic process, which deals with all aspects of CVD prevention. This includes the provision of dietary advice, antismoking measures and promotion of physical activity. Special attention should also be paid to treating hypertension and controlling diabetes. The first step in the management of dyslipidaemia is dietary intervention and the achievement of ideal body weight. The effectiveness of diet has recently received a boost with the introduction of functional foods; these include products containing plant stanol or sterol esters, consumption of which was endorsed by the latest NCEP guidelines.

The results of the Heart Protection Study has led to a marked increase in the use of statins by primary health care physicians. This in turn requires awareness of the target levels of LDL to be achieved and of the side-effects of these drugs. A final imperative is to evaluate and audit the completeness and success of all such interventions aimed at treating dyslipidaemia and preventing CVD.

1

Pathophysiology of plasma lipids

Introduction • Dyslipidaemia • The primary hypercholesterolaemias • The primary hypertriglyceridaemias • Primary mixed hyperlipidaemias • Secondary hyperlipidaemia • Primary hypolipoproteinaemia

INTRODUCTION

Simplification of the complex topic dealt with in this chapter is essential if it is to be read by non-specialists – but oversimplification carries its own risks. For example, the term 'cholesterol' includes both free (unesterified) cholesterol and cholesterol ester, which differ markedly in their physical properties, tissue distribution and physiological functions. Thus, two-thirds of the cholesterol in plasma is normally esterified by the enzyme lecithin cholesterol acyltransferase (LCAT), whereas in the rare inherited disorder due to deficiency of LCAT virtually all of the plasma cholesterol is free. Likewise, the extent to which cholesterol is transported in plasma within high density lipoprotein (HDL) as opposed to low density lipoprotein (LDL) is an important determinant of the propensity to develop atherosclerotic coronary heart disease (CHD). The lower the level of HDL cholesterol, the more likely it is that this disease will occur prematurely, even if the total cholesterol is within the normal range. The opposite applies to LDL cholesterol, increased levels predisposing to premature death from CHD, as exemplified by familial hypercholesterolaemia. Measuring total cholesterol alone does not differentiate between free and esterified cholesterol, nor between HDL and LDL.

What are lipids and what is their physiological role?

Lipids are fat-soluble compounds found in all living organisms. The three main species in humans are sterols, mainly cholesterol; glycerides, notably triglycerides, which consist of three fatty acid molecules esterified with glycerol; and phospholipids, mainly phosphatidyl choline (lecithin) and sphingomyelin.

Cholesterol is the best known lipid on account of its 'Jekyll and Hyde' characteristics of being both essential to life, as a constituent of cell membranes and precursor of steroid hormones, as well as being a crucial component of atherosclerosis, the commonest cause of death in countries like Britain and America. However, in quantitative terms, the mass of triglyceride transported in plasma greatly exceeds the amount of cholesterol. Oxidation of free fatty acids derived from hydrolysed triglyceride or released from adipose tissue provides a major source of energy for cardiac and skeletal muscle, especially during exercise. Although phospholipids are not measured routinely in clinical practice, this does not diminish their importance as key constituents of plasma lipoproteins and of the lipid bilayer which comprises all cell membranes.

Sterols, triglycerides and phospholipids can all be synthesized endogenously as well as ingested in the diet. However, essential ω-6 fatty acids and fat-soluble vitamins cannot be synthesized de novo and must be obtained from exogenous sources. Similarly, ω-3 fatty acids can only be obtained from marine and plant sources. Current evidence suggests that these long chain, polyunsaturated lipids have anti-arrhythmic properties and may also enhance neonatal brain development.

Cholesterol transport and metabolism

Much of what is known about lipid metabolism in health has resulted from studying inherited, often very rare defects of the pathways involved. In the light of such information, the main receptors and enzymes which regulate the synthesis, transport and catabolism of cholesterol and cholesterol-rich lipoproteins are now known, as shown schematically in Figure 1.1 To facilitate description the main sites involved have been divided into five physiological compartments.

Small intestine (jejunum and ileum)

Dietary and biliary cholesterol, totalling approximately 1 g/day, enter the duodenum via the pylorus and bile duct, respectively, and become incorporated into mixed micelles by the actions of pancreatic lipase and bile salts. Cholesterol absorption takes place in the jejunum via a highly specific mechanism which discriminates

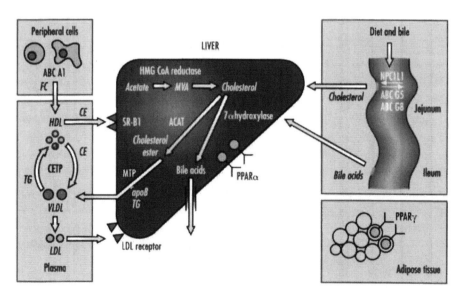

Figure 1.1 Schematic diagram of the major physiological compartments within and from which cholesterol is synthesized and secreted, transported and degraded. The enzymes, receptors and transfer proteins involved are shown (PPAR, peroxisome proliferator activated receptor; ACAT, acylcholesterol acyltransferase; MTP, microsomal triglyceride transfer protein; SR-B1, scavenger receptor class B, type 1; ABC A1, G5 and G8, ATP-binding cassette transporters A1, G5 and G8; NPC1L1, Niemann–Pick C1 Like 1 protein; CETP, cholesterol ester transfer protein).

between cholesterol, roughly half of which is absorbed, and plant sterols, which are absorbed only one-tenth as well, despite their close molecular similarity. Unabsorbed sterols undergo bacterial metabolism in the colon prior to excretion in the faeces.

During its transit through the intestinal mucosa much of the absorbed cholesterol is esterified by acylcholesterol acyltransferase (ACAT) before becoming incorporated into chylomicrons and entering the intestinal lymphatics, together with cholesterol synthesized by the intestine itself.

Once the lipid components of mixed micelles have been absorbed, the residual bile salts travel to the terminal ileum where they are efficiently re-absorbed via the sodium-dependent bile acid transporter (BAT) before entering the portal vein. Mutations of the BAT gene cause severe diarrhoea ('cholereic enteropathy').[1]

Liver

The liver is the major site of cholesterol synthesis and degradation. Synthesis is regulated by the enzyme hydroxymethyl glutaryl coenzyme A (HMGCoA) reductase, with conversion of acetate to mevalonic acid being the rate-limiting step. This reaction is under feedback regulation by its end product, cholesterol, including that entering the liver in chylomicron remnants and via the LDL receptor pathway. The latter is the main mechanism for the uptake and degradation of LDL, and LDL receptor activity is a key determinant of plasma cholesterol levels. Another determinant is the enzyme cholesterol 7α-hydroxylase, which mediates the conversion of cholesterol to bile acids. This reaction is under feedback regulation by reabsorbed bile acids returning to the liver via the portal vein. Interruption of the enterohepatic recycling of bile acids leads to an increased rate of conversion of cholesterol to bile acids via up-regulation of cholesterol 7α-hydroxylase and to an increased expression of LDL receptors, which decreases the level of LDL cholesterol in plasma.

Locally synthesized and recycled cholesterol entering the liver via the chylomicron remnant and LDL receptor pathways not only gets excreted in bile as bile acids, but is also secreted as biliary free cholesterol. Another route of secretion of cholesterol from the liver is into plasma as very low density lipoprotein (VLDL), although in this instance much of it undergoes preliminary esterification by the enzyme ACAT. The secretory process is also dependent upon microsomal triglyceride transfer protein (MTP), which mediates the incorporation of triglyceride and cholesterol ester within an outer shell of apolipoprotein B (apoB). Mutations of the MTP gene result in the rare disorder aβlipoproteinaemia, which is characterized by absence from plasma of cholesterol-carrying lipoproteins containing both forms of apoB, $apoB_{48}$ (chylomicrons) and $apoB_{100}$ (VLDL and LDL).

Plasma, peripheral cells and adipose tissue

As stated above, cholesterol is secreted into plasma mainly in VLDL particles which, as will be discussed later, undergo conversion into VLDL remnants and LDL. Prior to this, however, the composition of VLDL gets modified by cholesterol ester transfer protein (CETP), which exchanges triglyceride in VLDL for cholesterol ester in HDL. The cholesterol in HDL is acquired from peripheral cells such as monocytes and macrophages by a transfer mechanism that has recently been shown to be dependent upon the adenosine triphosphate (ATP)-binding cassette transporter

(ABC) A1, absence of which results in Tangier disease.[2] The free cholesterol acquired by HDL via this pathway is esterified by the enzyme LCAT and some of this cholesterol ester is then transferred to VLDL, as already mentioned. The remainder gets taken up by the liver via the so-called class B, type 1 scavenger receptor (SR-B1).[3]

Adipose tissue is predominantly involved in the metabolism of free fatty acids and their storage as triglyceride, but it also acts as a reservoir of free cholesterol and a source of CETP. Free fatty acids are ligands for peroxisome proliferator activated receptors (PPARs), which mediate oxidation of fatty acids in the liver (PPARα) and their storage as triglyceride in adipose tissue (PPARγ) respectively.[4]

Triglyceride transport and metabolism

The salient features of triglyceride transport, showing the precursor–product relationship between triglyceride-rich VLDL and cholesterol-rich LDL are illustrated in Figure 1.2.

Most of the fat in the diet is triglyceride, and more than 90% of this is absorbed following hydrolysis by pancreatic lipase and micellar solubilization by bile acids within the small intestine. The resultant free fatty acids and monoglycerides are resynthesized into triglyceride by enterocytes and then secreted as chylomicrons into intestinal lymph. Following entry into plasma both exogenous triglyceride in chylomicrons, as well as endogenously synthesized triglyceride secreted by the liver as VLDL, are subject to the action of the enzyme lipoprotein lipase, located in the walls of capillaries adjacent to skeletal muscle and adipose tissue. By hydrolysing triglyceride into free fatty acids and glycerol this enzyme converts chylomicrons and VLDL into chylomicron and VLDL remnants; the latter are sometimes termed intermediate density lipoprotein (IDL). Both types of remnant are taken up by the LDL and other receptors in the liver but a significant proportion of IDL is converted by hepatic lipase into LDL in plasma.

Free fatty acids released by the action of lipoprotein and hepatic lipases get taken up by adipose tissue for storage as triglyceride or for re-export into plasma bound to albumin. Subsequently, they are oxidized in skeletal muscle and the liver or converted by the latter to triglyceride and secreted back into plasma as VLDL.

Although not shown in Figure 1.2, the activity of lipoprotein lipase, and thus the efficiency of triglyceride-rich lipoprotein clearance, has an important influence on HDL metabolism. Several mechanisms are involved but the overall effect is that the slower the rate of removal of triglyceride, the lower the concentration of HDL cholesterol and vice versa. Thus, in most instances, hypertriglyceridaemia is associated with low levels of HDL cholesterol.

Factors influencing plasma lipids

The main constitutional influences on plasma lipids and lipoproteins are age and sex. In cord blood total cholesterol levels range from 1.65–2 mmol/L, distributed equally between LDL and HDL, with triglycerides in the region of 0.5 mmol/L. A rapid rise in cholesterol occurs during the first 6 months of life but there is little further change until after puberty, cholesterol and triglyceride values averaging approximately 4 and 0.65 mmol/L, respectively. After the age of 15 years, LDL cholesterol and triglyceride levels rise more in boys than girls and, unlike the latter,

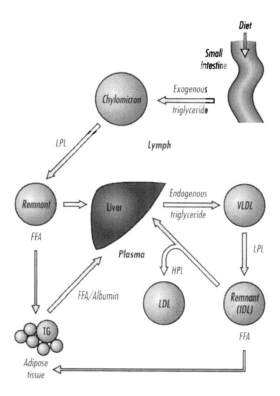

Figure 1.2 A simplified scheme of lipoprotein metabolism demonstrating the role of lipoprotein lipase (LPL) and hepatic lipase (HPL) in the conversion of triglyceride-rich chylomicrons and VLDL into free fatty acids (FFA) and cholesterol-rich chylomicron remnant particles, IDL and LDL. Adipose tissue takes up and stores FFA as triglyceride (TG), which is then released back into plasma bound to albumin.

their HDL cholesterol falls, reflecting the opposite effects of androgens and oestrogens.

The main life-style influences on plasma lipids are diet, exercise, seasonal variation and intercurrent illness. Saturated fats raise and polyunsaturated fats lower LDL cholesterol, whereas excessive intake of carbohydrate and obesity increase triglyceride levels and lower HDL cholesterol. In contrast, exercise lowers triglyceride and raises HDL cholesterol, whereas alcohol increases both.

Day-to-day fluctuations in serum cholesterol range from 5–10%, roughly half of which reflects analytical variation. Recent food intake has little effect on serum cholesterol, whereas triglycerides rise markedly after a meal. Both lipids tend to be lower in summer than winter.

Intercurrent disease can influence serum lipids acutely, as occurs after a myocardial infarct. There is a 24-h window of opportunity for measuring serum lipids following such an event, after which cholesterol levels fall and triglycerides rise, these changes persisting for several weeks. Underlying malignant disease sometimes manifests itself as an unexpected and sustained decrease in serum cholesterol.

DYSLIPIDAEMIA

Definition, classification and prevalence

The term dyslipidaemia encompasses abnormalities of lipoprotein transport associated with a decrease of lipids in plasma, hypolipidaemia, as well as those causing an excess, hyperlipidaemia. The definition of dyslipidaemia has gradually evolved as a result of advances in the understanding of the underlying mechanisms. Many monogenically-inherited disorders can now be defined in terms of the specific mutation(s) responsible for encoding the dysfunctional receptor, ligand or enzyme causing dyslipidaemia, whereas most polygenic and secondary forms of dyslipidaemia are still defined by arbitrary cut-offs such as the 5th and 95th percentile of the distribution of the lipid or lipoprotein variable in question.

In a similar manner the classification of dyslipidaemia has evolved from the Fredrickson and World Health Organization classifications of lipoprotein phenotypes devised over 30 years ago to the simpler system now in use. This includes both hypolipidaemia and hyperlipidaemia and differentiates the latter into hypercholesterolaemia, hypertriglyceridaemia and mixed hyperlipidaemia.

The prevalence of the major genetically-determined forms of dyslipidaemia predisposing to premature CHD are shown in Table 1.1. The frequency of polygenic hypercholesterolaemia is based on the premise that it is responsible for all serum cholesterol levels above the 95th percentile not accounted for by familial hypercholesterolaemia (FH), familial defective apoB$_{100}$ (FDB) or familial combined hyperlipidaemia (FCH). The prevalence of FH is increased in parts of the world where an imported founder gene effect has been operative, such as South Africa and French Canada.

Table 1.1 Estimated prevalence of inherited forms of dyslipidaemia predisposing to atherosclerosis

Disorder	Phenotype	Prevalence
Familial hypercholesterolaemia	VLDL remnants and LDL increased	2 : 1000
Familial defective apoB$_{100}$	LDL increased	1 : 1000
Familial combined hyperlipidaemia	VLDL or LDL or both increased	5 : 1000
Type III hyperlipoproteinaemia	Chylomicron and VLDL remnants increased	0.1 : 1000
Polygenic hypercholesterolaemia	LDL moderately increased	42 : 1000
Familial hypoalipoproteinaemia	HDL decreased	50 : 1000

VLDL, very low density lipoprotein; LDL, low density lipoprotein; apoB$_{100}$, apolipoprotein B; HDL, high density lipoprotein.

Reproduced with permission from Thompson G, Abnormalities of plasma lipoprotein transport. In Barter PJ, Rye K-A: *Plasma lipids and their role in disease*. © 1999 Harwood Academic Publishers, Australia.

THE PRIMARY HYPERCHOLESTEROLAEMIAS

These comprise several disorders resulting from increases in LDL or HDL known or presumed to be genetic in origin in the absence of any cause of secondary hypercholesterolaemia. This section also includes genetic disorders characterized by the accumulation in plasma and tissues of abnormal amounts of other sterols, notably plant sterols (phytosterolaemia) and cholestanol (cerebro-tendinous xanthomatosis), and also cholesterol ester storage disease.

Familial hypercholesterolaemia (FH)

This disorder affects approximately 0.2% of the population (see Table 1.1) and is usually due to dominant inheritance of a mutant gene encoding the LDL receptor (heterozygous FH), or rarely to inheritance of two mutant alleles (homozygous FH). To date more than 900 distinct mutations of the LDL receptor gene have been described.[5]

Deficient expression or defective function of LDL receptors in FH results in accumulation of LDL, causing hypercholesterolaemia from birth. Serum total cholesterol ranges between 8 and 15 mmol/L in adult heterozygotes and between 15 and 30 mmol/L in homozygotes. Triglyceride levels are usually normal in affected children, but a moderately raised triglyceride is not uncommon in adults. HDL cholesterol is normal or reduced.

A definitive diagnosis of FH depends upon identifying the mutant gene or demonstrating a deficiency of LDL receptors in fresh or cultured cells. However, the presence of tendon xanthomas in a hypercholesterolaemic individual, or a raised LDL cholesterol in someone with a hypercholesterolaemic first-degree relative with tendon xanthomas, is presumptive proof of heterozygous FH.

Homozygous FH, which often results from consanguineous unions between heterozygotes, is a rare condition characterized by extreme hypercholesterolaemia and the early onset of cutaneous planar or tuberose xanthomas, tendon xanthomas and corneal arcus. Atheromatous involvement of the aortic root is evident by puberty, manifested by an aortic systolic murmur, and coronary ostial stenosis commonly leads to sudden death during early adulthood. A milder form, known as autosomal recessive hypercholesterolaemia, results from recessively inherited mutations of the ARH gene.[6]

Heterozygous FH may be detected early when screening an affected family but often remains undiagnosed until the onset of cardiovascular symptoms in adult life. There is a marked increase in the risk of premature CHD in both males and females.[7] In addition to hypercholesterolaemia, heterozygotes may show external signs of cholesterol deposition, such as corneal arcus, xanthelasma and tendon xanthomas (see Chapter 5), indicative of underlying atherosclerosis (Figure 1.3).

It has been estimated that the onset of CHD occurs about 20 years earlier in those with FH than in the remainder of the population. One factor influencing the presence of vascular disease is the HDL cholesterol, high levels being protective; another factor is smoking, the age of onset of CHD in women with FH who smoke being similar to that in men. On angiography, over 70% of male heterozygotes have triple vessel disease and one-third have disease of the left main stem. An unusually severe form of heterozygous FH can be caused by missense mutations of the PCSK9 gene.[8]

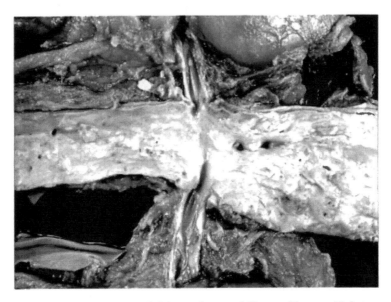

Figure 1.3 Severe atherosclerosis of abdominal aorta of 40-year-old man with heterozygous familial hypercholesterolaemia who died suddenly from myocardial infarction.

Familial defective apoB$_{100}$

This inherited disorder, often abbreviated to FDB, is caused by a single amino acid substitution (glutamine for arginine) at residue 3500 in apoB.[9] This results in an almost complete loss of ability of LDL to bind to its receptor. Estimates of frequency vary, but FDB is probably about half as common as FH. Affected individuals usually have moderate hypercholesterolaemia, but some heterozygotes present with clinical features which are indistinguishable from FH.

Polygenic hypercholesterolaemia

Plasma cholesterol levels are under the control of many different genes and environmental factors, the summated effects of which give a near-Gaussian distribution of cholesterol levels in the population. The clustering in an individual and within families of several genes which together induce moderate elevations of plasma cholesterol is termed polygenic or sporadic hypercholesterolaemia.

Polygenic hypercholesterolaemia lacks the classical clinical features of FH but does appear to be associated with premature atherosclerosis. Estimates of the prevalence of polygenic hypercholesterolaemia vary according to the criterion used to define the upper limit of normal for serum cholesterol. Obviously, the lower the cut-off value used the higher will be its estimated frequency in the population.

Familial hyperαlipoproteinaemia

Hyperαlipoproteinaemia, defined as an HDL cholesterol >2mmol/L, sometimes occurs on a familial basis. Familial hyperαlipoproteinaemia is a heterogeneous entity in that some families show a clear-cut autosomal dominant pattern of inheritance, while in others the features suggest interaction between polygenic influences and common environmental factors within the household, such as alcohol. The syndrome often tends to be associated with a decreased frequency of CHD and with longevity. However, groups of patients have been described in Japan and elsewhere with familial hyperalipoproteinaemia due to a deficiency of CETP activity in plasma; such individuals sometimes develop CHD despite their high HDL.[10]

Cholesterol ester storage disease

A rare cause of primary hypercholesterolaemia is inherited deficiency of cholesterol ester hydrolase, which gives rise to cholesterol ester storage disease. Mutations of this lysosomal enzyme[11] impair hydrolysis of cholesterol ester, resulting in a failure of down-regulation of HMG CoA reductase. In plasma, LDL cholesterol is increased whereas HDL cholesterol is reduced. Clinically the disorder is characterized by hepatic and splenic enlargement but xanthomas are absent. Treatment with an HMG CoA reductase inhibitor lowers LDL cholesterol and may prevent the accelerated atherosclerosis which has been described in this disorder.

Phytosterolaemia (sitosterolaemia)

This recessively inherited disorder is characterized by excessive absorption of plant sterols, manifested by an increase in plasma levels of sitosterol and campesterol. This is accompanied by a moderate increase in LDL cholesterol and the early onset of tendon xanthomas and atherosclerosis. The underlying genetic defect has recently been identified as mutations in either of two tandem ATP-binding cassette (ABC) transporter genes, ABC G5 and ABC G8.[12] Intestinal uptake of cholesterol and plant sterols from mixed micelles is mediated by Niemann–Pick C1 Like 1 (NPC1L1) protein, located in the brush border of enterocytes.[13] Under normal circumstances ABC G5 and G8 actively promote efflux back into the intestinal lumen of most of the plant sterol taken up via the NPC1L1 pathway, while permitting the influx of 40–50% of the cholesterol. In patients with mutations of ABC G5 and G8 this mechanism is defective, resulting in hyperabsorption of both cholesterol and plant sterols. Affected individuals respond well to treatment with ezetimibe, which blocks uptake of cholesterol and plant sterols via NPC1L1 and reduces plasma levels of both.

Cerebro-tendinous xanthomatosis

This rare, recessively inherited disorder is characterized by tendon xanthomas, cataracts and neurological dysfunction. The disease is due to mutations affecting sterol 27α-hydroxylase,[14] an enzyme involved in the conversion of cholesterol to bile acids. Deficiency results in accumulation of cholestanol in plasma and tissues, notably the central nervous system and tendons. Untreated these patients develop dementia and are at increased risk of premature atherosclerosis.

Hyperlipoprotein(a)aemia

Lipoprotein(a), or Lp(a), consists of an LDL particle covalently linked to a molecule of apolipoprotein(a). The latter is polymorphic and at least 34 isoforms have been described,[15] which vary markedly in size. The distribution of Lp(a) in Caucasian populations is skewed, high plasma levels being associated with low molecular weight isoforms of apo(a). The inverse correlation between Lp(a) concentration in plasma and particle size is explained by higher rates of secretion of smaller isoforms.

The importance of Lp(a) as a risk factor for cardiovascular disease remains controversial. Case–control studies have suggested that risk increases with Lp(a) levels above 30 mg/dl, whereas in a large prospective study the risk of myocardial infarction increased steeply only above 60 mg/dl.[16] No studies have been done which show therapeutic benefit from lowering Lp(a) per se, but reduction of concomitant increases in LDL cholesterol appears to reduce the risk associated with a raised Lp(a).[17]

THE PRIMARY HYPERTRIGLYCERIDAEMIAS

This section considers disorders characterized by predominant hypertriglyceridaemia resulting from increases in fasting plasma of chylomicrons and/or VLDL without any obvious secondary cause. Evidence of the hereditary basis of some of these disorders is often presumptive in the absence of genetic markers.

Familial lipoprotein lipase deficiency

This rare disorder, also known as familial type I hyperlipoproteinaemia, is characterized by marked hypertriglyceridaemia and chylomicronaemia, and usually presents in childhood. It is due to homozygous or compound heterozygous inheritance of mutations of the gene for lipoprotein lipase.[18] Complete or subtotal deficiency of the enzyme ensues and results in a failure of lipolysis and accumulation of chylomicrons in plasma. The main clinical features are recurrent episodes of abdominal pain, often resembling acute pancreatitis, eruptive xanthomas, hepatosplenomegaly and lipaemia retinalis, associated with serum triglycerides in the region of 50–100 mmol/L.

There seems to be no increased susceptibility to atherosclerosis in this condition. Gross chylomicronaemia results in a marked increase in serum cholesterol as well as triglyceride. The diagnosis depends upon demonstrating that plasma lipoprotein lipase levels are less than 10% of normal following an intravenous dose of heparin 5000 iu.

Heterozygous carriers occur with a frequency of 1 : 500 and tend to have higher triglyceride and apoB levels and lower levels of HDL cholesterol and post-heparin lipolytic activity (PHLA) than their unaffected relatives. These features suggest that, unlike homozygotes, heterozygotes may be at increased risk of CHD.[19]

Familial apoC-II deficiency

This disorder is due to recessively inherited mutations of the gene for apoC-II which result in defective lipolysis and hypertriglyceridaemia. Lipoprotein lipase is present in normal amounts but cannot hydrolyse chylomicrons or VLDL in the absence of normal apoC-II, which activates the enzyme in plasma.

Homozygotes have triglycerides in the range of 15–107 mmol/L and often develop acute pancreatitis. Premature vascular disease is unusual but has been described. Heterozygotes exhibit a 30–50% decrease in apoC-II levels and a tendency to raised triglycerides.[20] A similar syndrome has been described recently in association with apolipoprotein A-V deficiency.

Familial hypertriglyceridaemia

This disorder is subdivided according to whether the predominant abnormality in affected individuals is an excess of VLDL alone (type IV) or plus an excess of chylomicrons (type V). However, there is some overlap within families and it is probable that similar genetic abnormalities are responsible for both varieties of the disorder, with a more severe expression in those with a type V phenotype.

Familial type IV hyperlipoproteinaemia is characterized by moderate hypertriglyceridaemia due to increased levels of VLDL, with an autosomal dominant pattern of inheritance. The frequency of the disorder in the adult population has been estimated at 0.2–0.3%, but it is expressed less frequently in childhood. Fasting values of serum cholesterol and triglyceride averaged 6.2 and 3.0 mmol/L, respectively, in one series of patients.

Affected patients have larger than normal VLDL particles with an increased triglyceride:apoB ratio, accompanied by a decrease in HDL cholesterol. Free fatty acid flux into triglyceride is raised, which is accompanied by an increase in VLDL synthesis and a decrease in the proportion of VLDL converted to LDL.

The underlying mechanism for the overproduction of VLDL triglyceride remains to be determined but insulin resistance may be involved. Administration of corticosteroids or oestrogens accentuates the hypertriglyceridaemia and can lead to acute pancreatitis. Recent data suggest that the risk of myocardial infarction is increased.[21]

Familial type V hyperlipoproteinaemia is an uncommon disorder characterized by an increase in both VLDL and chylomicrons; the hypertriglyceridaemia is accentuated by obesity and alcohol consumption. Unlike type I hyperlipoproteinaemia it seldom presents in childhood, and post-heparin lipoprotein lipase and hepatic lipase activities are usually normal. However, there is a similar liability to develop acute pancreatitis. Other features are eruptive xanthomas, glucose intolerance, hyperuricaemia and peripheral neuropathy.

PRIMARY MIXED HYPERLIPIDAEMIAS

Under this heading come disorders with little in common other than the presence of concomitant hypertriglyceridaemia and hypercholesterolaemia.

Familial combined hyperlipidaemia (FCH)

This entity was first described in hyperlipidaemic patients who survived a myocardial infarction and had elevations of both cholesterol and triglyceride. Roughly 50% of their relatives were hyperlipidaemic, of whom a third had hypercholesterolaemia (type IIa), a third had hypertriglyceridaemia (type IV or V) and a third had both abnormalities (type IIb). Opinions differ as to whether the mode of inheritance is monogenic or polygenic but current evidence favours the latter explanation. Whatever its mode of inheritance FCH is a relatively common disorder, occurring in up to 0.5% of the general population. It differs from FH in that affected children are never hypercholesterolaemic, hypertriglyceridaemia being the earliest manifestation of the disorder, and differs from familial hypertriglyceridaemia in that the latter is never associated with an elevated LDL cholesterol.

Although the nature of the genetic defect is unknown, the disorder is characterized by increased secretion of apoB$_{100}$, both as VLDL and LDL,[22] resulting in raised plasma apoB levels. Other metabolic abnormalities ascribed to FCH include insulin resistance, raised free fatty acid levels, delayed chylomicron remnant clearance and partial deficiency of lipoprotein lipase. There seems to be no evidence of a defect of the apoB gene to explain the overproduction of apoB.

There are no distinctive clinical features in FCH and the diagnosis depends upon family studies. Cabezas et al[23] have proposed the following criteria for diagnosing FCH: the presence of primary hyperlipidaemia, with a serum cholesterol of >6.5 mmol/L and/or triglyceride >2 mmol/L and an apoB >90 mg/dl in the patient; at least one first degree relative with a different lipoprotein phenotype; and a history of coronary or cerebrovascular disease in a first or second degree relative before the age of 60 years. The condition is undoubtedly associated with an increased risk of atherosclerosis and CHD.[21]

Type III hyperlipoproteinaemia

This disorder, also known as familial dysbetalipoproteinaemia, is characterized by the accumulation in plasma of chylomicron and VLDL remnants. Under normal circumstances these particles are taken up by hepatic receptors which recognize the apolipoprotein E on their surface, normally either $apoE_3$ or E_4. However, particles containing $apoE_2$, in which there is substitution of cysteine for arginine at position 158, show virtually no binding to these receptors and fail to get cleared at a normal rate.[24] Most patients with type III hyperlipoproteinaemia are homozygous for $apoE_2$, but in some it is due to inheritance of rarer variants.

The commonest mutation behaves in a recessive manner and affected individuals (frequency 1:100) develop overt type III hyperlipoproteinaemia (frequency 1:10,000) only if additional factors are present. These either reduce the number of receptors expressed (such as FH and hypothyroidism) or enhance the rate of secretion of VLDL and thereby increase the number of remnants generated by lipolysis (e.g. non-insulin-dependent diabetes mellitus). Similarly, a high-fat diet promotes chylomicron-remnant formation. Hormonal influences are also important in that recessive type III hyperlipidaemia seldom presents in males before puberty or in females before the menopause.

Clinical features of type III include corneal arcus, xanthelasma, tubero-eruptive xanthomas on knees and elbows and, pathognomonically, palmar striae (see Chapter 5). Serum cholesterol and triglyceride are both elevated, usually to about 10 mmol/L, and lipoprotein electrophoresis shows the 'broad β' band characteristic of remnant particles. The diagnosis should be confirmed by apoE genotyping or phenotyping. LDL cholesterol is reduced because of decreased conversion of IDL to LDL but, despite this, atherosclerosis is common and presumably reflects the atherogenic properties of the remnant particles. Vascular disease occurs in over 50% of patients, involving not only the coronary tree, but also peripheral and cerebral vessels. Glucose intolerance and hyperuricaemia are common and acute pancreatitis can also occur.

Familial hepatic lipase deficiency

This rare form of mixed dyslipidaemia has many of the features of type III hyperlipoproteinaemia, including accumulation of remnant particles. However, the underlying cause is unrelated to apoE polymorphism but is due to mutations of the gene for hepatic lipase, which under normal circumstances mediates the conversion of IDL to LDL.

SECONDARY HYPERLIPIDAEMIA

Hyperlipidaemia can be secondary to a number of diseases, hormonal disturbances and iatrogenic agents.

Hormonal influences

Pregnancy

Pregnancy is normally accompanied by moderate rises in cholesterol and triglyceride reflecting increases in VLDL, LDL and HDL, due to the increase in oestrogens. Marked rises in cholesterol are usual in FH during pregnancy, which can also markedly exacerbate pre-existing hypertriglyceridaemia, especially when this is due to lipoprotein lipase deficiency.

Exogenous sex hormones

Oral contraceptive use seems to be associated with increased levels of total and HDL cholesterol and triglycerides. Hormone replacement therapy with oestrogen alone or combined with progestogen is associated with increases in HDL cholesterol and triglyceride and decreases in LDL cholesterol and Lp(a). So far there is no evidence that these effects have had any impact, one way or another, on CHD mortality.

Rarely, oral oestrogens, whether given as a contraceptive or replacement therapy, or for the treatment of prostatic cancer, have caused marked hypertriglyceridaemia and acute pancreatitis.

Hypothyroidism

Hypothyroidism has long been recognized as an important and relatively common cause of hyperlipidaemia. Usually this presents as hypercholesterolaemia due to an increase in LDL that was caused by a decrease in receptor-mediated catabolism. It is reversible by replacement therapy with L-thyroxine.

Metabolic disorders

Diabetes mellitus

Untreated juvenile onset, type I or insulin-dependent diabetes mellitus (IDDM) is accompanied by marked hypertriglyceridaemia, due partly to deficiency of lipoprotein lipase consequent on insulin lack and partly to an increased flux of free fatty acids from adipose tissue, which promotes hepatic triglyceride synthesis.

Maturity onset, type II or non-insulin-dependent diabetes mellitus (NIDDM) is often associated with obesity and is characterized by insulin resistance. The commonest lipid abnormality is hypertriglyceridaemia, due mainly to increased production of large VLDL particles. Clearance of triglyceride is also impaired owing to decreased lipoprotein lipase activity, but the proportion of VLDL converted to LDL is decreased, so that LDL levels are often normal.

Gout

Hypertriglyceridaemia is a common accompaniment of gout but there appears to be no direct metabolic link between hyperuricaemia and hypertriglyceridaemia. The association may simply reflect the fact that obesity, use of alcohol and administration of thiazides are common to both.

Obesity

Hypertriglyceridaemia, glucose intolerance, hyperinsulinism and vascular disease all commonly accompany obesity. HDL cholesterol is low, being inversely correlated with body weight, but its level rises with weight reduction. Total cholesterol and LDL levels are often normal but turnover studies show an increased rate of cholesterol synthesis.

These metabolic abnormalities are especially common in association with the central or abdominal pattern of obesity, which has been shown to be an independent risk factor for cardiovascular mortality in middle-aged men.[25]

Renal dysfunction

Hyperlipidaemia, often severe, is common in the nephrotic syndrome. Hypoalbuminaemia appears to play a central role, probably by diverting increased amounts of free fatty acids to the liver and thus stimulating apoB secretion. LDL cholesterol is inversely correlated with serum albumin and is often markedly raised, as too are Lp(a) levels. Accelerated vascular disease can be a major consequence of persistent hyperlipidaemia in such patients.

Hyperlipidaemia is common also in patients with chronic renal failure, but in contrast to the nephrotic syndrome, hypertriglyceridaemia is much commoner than hypercholesterolaemia. This appears to be secondary to impaired lipolysis, possibly because of inhibition of lipoprotein lipase by a non-dialysable factor present in uraemic plasma. Increased concentrations of remnant particles and decreases in HDL cholesterol occur in patients with chronic renal failure, including those on haemodialysis. Lp(a) levels are increased two to fourfold in patients on haemodialysis.[26] Dyslipidaemia predicts the likelihood of CHD, a common cause of death in such patients.[27]

Hyperlipidaemia also appears to be common in patients on chronic ambulatory peritoneal dialysis (CAPD), but the pattern differs from that seen with haemodialysis, possibly reflecting the absence of heparin administration in CAPD. Hyperlipidaemia often persists after successful renal transplantation, and immunosuppressive drugs probably play an important role, especially steroids.

Obstructive liver disease

Primary biliary cirrhosis or prolonged cholestasis from other causes is accompanied by marked hyperlipidaemia, resulting from reflux of biliary lecithin and free cholesterol into plasma. Xanthelasma can be a prominent accompaniment of the hypercholesterolaemia of primary biliary cirrhosis.

Beverages

Excessive consumption of ethanol is a common cause of secondary hypertriglyceri-daemia, especially in males. Even moderate consumption of alcohol on a regular basis results in significantly higher serum triglyceride levels than are found in total abstainers. Withdrawal of alcohol results in a rapid decrease in triglyceride levels.

An increased level of HDL cholesterol is an even commoner consequence of heavy consumption of alcohol than is hypertriglyceridaemia and reflects the increase in lipoprotein lipase activity in adipose tissue which accompanies regular drinking, as opposed to the increase of that enzyme in skeletal muscle with exercise.

Frequent consumption of boiled or percolated coffee can result in increases in serum cholesterol and triglyceride. These effects are mediated by diterpenes contained in oils leached out from coffee beans but the mechanism is unclear.[28]

Iatrogenic effects

Administration of thiazide diuretics such as chlorthalidone and hydrochlorothiazide has long been recognized to increase total cholesterol and triglyceride. HDL cholesterol changes little but VLDL and LDL cholesterols both increase. These changes probably reflect the adverse effects of these drugs on glucose tolerance.

Long-term administration of β-blockers without intrinsic sympathomimetic activity (ISA) is associated with increases in serum triglyceride and decreases in HDL cholesterol; β-blockers with ISA have a much less marked influence on serum triglyceride and, like α-blockers, cause an increase in HDL cholesterol.

Immunosuppressive doses of corticosteroids cause insulin resistance and impaired glucose tolerance, which leads to hypertriglyceridaemia and a reduction in HDL cholesterol. Experimental studies suggest that a steroid-induced increase in VLDL synthesis is responsible.

Studies in renal transplant patients on cyclosporin showed that this drug causes an increase in serum cholesterol, reflecting an increase in LDL cholesterol. It has been suggested that the latter reflects a hepatotoxic effect of the drug, which impairs receptor-mediated LDL catabolism.

An increase in HDL cholesterol has been well documented in epileptic patients receiving phenytoin, and a similar effect has been reported with cimetidine but not ranitidine. Retinoids induce a marked increase in serum triglycerides, especially in patients with pre-existing hypertriglyceridaemia. Amiodarone can cause hyper-cholesterolaemia independently of its effects on thyroid function. Antiretroviral therapy for HIV infections is becoming an increasingly common cause of iatrogenic dyslipidaemia.

PRIMARY HYPOLIPOPROTEINAEMIA

Aβlipoproteinaemia

This rare, recessively inherited disease is characterized by the onset during infancy of malabsorption and anaemia accompanied by the development in later childhood of progressively severe ataxia and retinitis pigmentosa. Plasma is lacking in chylomicrons, VLDL and LDL. Serum cholesterol and triglyceride levels are both very low, usually in the range 0.5–2 mmol/L, and apoB is undetectable. Nearly all the cholesterol in plasma is present as HDL.

The majority of patients described are males and result from consanguineous unions. Obligate heterozygotes show no signs of disease and have normal serum lipids. Homozygotes usually present with steatorrhoea in early childhood and jejunal biopsy shows the characteristic lipid-filled villi; the liver too contains excess fat. The disorder is due to mutations of the gene encoding microsomal triglyceride transfer protein (MTP), which is essential for the incorporation of non-polar lipids into apoB-containing lipoproteins, and for secretion of the latter by the liver and small intestine.[29]

Malabsorption of fat-soluble vitamins can lead to osteomalacia but deficiency of vitamin D is less common than that of vitamins A, E and K. Aβlipoproteinaemia represents the most severe vitamin E deficiency state known in humans, but vitamin E supplementation prevents the development of neurological symptoms if given in childhood.

Familial hypoβlipoproteinaemia

The homozygous form of this disorder presents in a manner either identical to or as a milder version of aβlipoproteinaemia. It differs in that heterozygotes have LDL levels that are only 25% of normal. Thus the disorder appears to be inherited in an autosomal dominant manner and results from mutations of the apoB gene, the severity of clinical manifestations correlating inversely with the amount of apoB synthesized.[30]

Familial hypoαlipoproteinaemia

ApoA-I mutations

Familial absence or deficiency of HDL is a relatively rare disorder which is usually due to either Tangier disease, familial deficiency of lecithin cholesterol acyltransferase (LCAT) or mutations of the apoA-I gene,[31] apoA-I being the major apolipoprotein of HDL. Most apoA-I mutations are silent but a minority are associated with HDL deficiency. Clinical features associated with such mutations include corneal opacities, xanthomas and premaure CHD.

In a recent survey 10% of individuals with hypoαlipoproteinaemia were found to have a dysfunctional mutation of lipoprotein lipase.[32] However, familial hypoαlipoproteinaemia has also been reported in the absence of any detectable abnormality of apoA-I, lipoprotein lipase or LCAT.

Tangier disease

Tangier disease is a rare disorder characterized by hypocholesterolaemia, with enlargement of liver, spleen, lymph nodes and orange-coloured tonsils. Histology reveals the presence in these organs of numerous macrophages containing cholesterol ester, or foam cells, and an almost complete absence of HDL in plasma. Peripheral neuropathy is a common complication and there is an increased frequency of cardiovascular disease in middle age.[33] Recently it has been shown that Tangier disease results from mutations of the ABC A1 gene, with a consequent defect in the efflux of cholesterol from cells to HDL.[2]

Secondary hypolipoproteinaemia

Hypocholesterolaemia can occur secondary to malabsorption, with decreases in both LDL and HDL cholesterol in the face of normal or increased levels of VLDL. Patients with steatorrhoea have reduced amounts of linoleic acid in their plasma and clinical essential fatty acid deficiency has been documented in such individuals.

Hypocholesterolaemia can be induced surgically by ileal resection or by creating a partial ileal bypass. Both procedures lower LDL levels by preventing reabsorption of bile acids, which stimulates receptor-mediated LDL catabolism.

REFERENCES

1. Small DM. Point mutations in the ileal bile salt transporter cause leaks in the enterohepatic circulation leading to severe chronic diarrhoea and malabsorption. J Clin Invest 1997; 99:1807–8.
2. Young SG, Fielding CJ. The ABCs of cholesterol efflux. Nat Genet 1999; 22:316–18.
3. Krieger M. The 'best' of cholesterols, the 'worst' of cholesterols: a tale of two receptors. Proc Natl Acad Sci USA 1998; 95:4077–80.
4. Staels B, Koenig V, Habib A et al. Activation of human aortic smooth muscle cells is inhibited by PPARα but not by PPARγ activators. Nature 1998; 393:790–2.
5. Rader DJ, Cohen J, Hobbs H. Monogenic hypercholesterolemia: new insights in pathogenesis and treatment. J Clin Invest 2003; 111:1795–803.
6. Naoumova RP, Neuwirth C, Lee P et al. Autosomal recessive hypercholesterolaemia: long-term follow up and response to treatment. Atherosclerosis 2004; 274:165–72.
7. Scientific Steering Committee on behalf of the Simon Broome Register Group. Risk of fatal coronary heart disease in familial hypercholesterolaemia. Br Med J 1991; 303:893–6.
8. Sun XM, Eden ER, Tosi I et al. Evidence for effect of mutant PCSK9 on apolipoprotein B secretion as the cause of unusually severe dominant hypercholesterolaemia. Hum Mol Genet 2005; 14:1161–9.
9. Innerarity TL, Mahley RW, Weisgraber KH et al. Familial defective apolipoprotein B-100: a mutation of apolipoprotein B that causes hypercholesterolemia. J Lipid Res 1990; 31:1337–49.
10. Thompson GR. Is good cholesterol always good? Br Med J 2004; 329:471–2.
11. Ameis D, Brockmann G, Knoblich R et al. A 5′ splice-region mutation and a dinucleotide deletion in the lysosomal acid lipase gene in two patients with cholesteryl ester storage disease. J Lipid Res 1995; 36:241–50.
12. Lee MH, Lu K, Patel SB. Genetic basis of sitosterolaemia. Curr Opin Lipidol 2001; 12:141–9.
13. Altmann SW, Davis HR Jr, Zhu L-J et al. Niemann–Pick C1 Like 1 protein is critical for intestinal cholesterol absorption. Science 2004; 303:1201–4.
14. Kim KS, Kubota S, Kuriyama M et al. Identification of new mutations in sterol 27-hydroxylase gene in Japanese patients with cerebrotendinous xanthomatosis (CTX). J Lipid Res 1994; 35:1031–9.
15. Marcovina SM, Zhang ZZH, Gaur VP et al. Identification of 34 apolipoprotein(a) isoforms: differential expression of apolipoprotein(a) alleles between American blacks and whites. Biochem Biophys Res Commun 1993; 191:1192–6.
16. Cremer P, Nagel D, Labrot B et al. Lipoprotein Lp(a) as predictor of myocardial infarction in comparison to fibrinogen, LDL cholesterol and other risk factors: results from the prospective Gottingen Risk Incidence and Prevalence Study (GRIPS). Eur J Clin Invest 1994; 24:444–53.
17. Thompson GR, Maher VMG, Matthews S et al. Familial hypercholesterolaemia regression study: a randomised trial of low-density-lipoprotein apheresis. Lancet 1995; 345:811–16.
18. Hayden M, Ma Y, Brunzell J et al. Genetic variants affecting human lipoprotein and hepatic lipases. Curr Opin Lipidol 1991; 2:104–9.

19. Bijvoet S, Gagne SE, Moorjani S et al. Alterations in plasma lipoproteins and apolipoproteins before the age of 40 in heterozygotes for lipoprotein lipase deficiency. J Lipid Res 1996; 37:640–50.
20. Santamarina-Fojo S. Genetic dyslipoproteinemias: role of lipoprotein lipase and apolipoprotein C-II. Curr Opin Lipidol 1992; 3:186–95.
21. Hopkins PN, Heiss G, Ellison RC et al. Coronary artery disease risk in familial combined hyperlipidemia and familial hypertriglyceridemia: a case–control comparison from the National Heart, Lung and Blood Institute Family Heart Study. Circulation 2003; 108:519–23.
22. Grundy SM, Chait A, Brunzell JD. Familial combined hyperlipidaemia workshop. Arteriosclerosis 1987; 7:203–7.
23. Cabezas MC, de Bruin TWA, de Valk HW et al. Impaired fatty acid metabolism in familial combined hyperlipidemia. A mechanism associating hepatic apolipoprotein B overproduction and insulin resistance. J Clin Invest 1993; 92:160–8.
24. Mahley RW, Innerarity TL, Rall SC et al. Plasma lipoproteins: apolipoprotein structure and function. J Lipid Res 1984; 25:1277–94.
25. Kannel WB, Cupples LA, Ramaswami R et al. Regional obesity and risk of cardiovascular disease; the Framingham Study. J Clin Epidemiol 1991; 44:183–90.
26. Dieplinger H, Lackner C, Kronenberg F et al. Elevated plasma concentrations of lipoprotein(a) in patients with end-stage renal disease are not related to the size polymorphism of apolipoprotein(a). J Clin Invest 1993; 91:397–401.
27. Tschope W, Koch M, Thomas B et al. Serum lipids predict cardiac death in diabetic patients on maintenance hemodialysis. Results of a prospective study. The German Study Group Diabetes and Uremia. Nephron 1993; 64:354–8.
28. Mensink RP, Lebbink WJ, Lobbezoo IE et al. Diterpene composition of oils from Arabica and Robusta coffee beans and their effects on serum lipids in man. J Intern Med 1995; 237:543–50.
29. Sharp D, Blinderman L, Combs KA et al. Cloning and gene defects in microsomal triglyceride transfer protein associated with abetalipoproteinaemia. Nature 1993; 365:65–9.
30. Innerarity TL. Familial apolipoprotein B100: genetic disorders associated with apolipoprotein B. Curr Opin Lipidol 1990; 1:104–9.
31. Funke H. Genetic determinants of high density lipoprotein levels. Curr Opin Lipidol 1997; 8:189–96.
32. Reymer PW, Gagne E, Groenemeyer BE et al. A lipoprotein lipase mutation (Asn291Ser) is associated with reduced HDL cholesterol levels in premature atherosclerosis. Nat Genet 1995; 10:28–34.
33. Serfaty Lacrosniere C, Civeira F, Lanzberg A et al. Homozygous Tangier disease and cardiovascular disease. Atherosclerosis 1994; 107; 85–98.

2

Dyslipidaemia as a risk factor for cardiovascular disease

Introduction • National and regional differences • Age, gender and racial differences
• Type of risk • Trends in coronary heart disease

INTRODUCTION

While clinical dyslipidaemias have a biochemical basis and characteristic signs, symptoms and laboratory findings, a population-based perspective offers another view. In the early 1900s adults infrequently lived past the age of 50 years, chronic diseases were uncommon, and acute infections accounted for most deaths. The advent of antimicrobial agents and widespread use of immunization led to greatly improved control of acute and chronic infections by the middle of the 20th century. Faced with an ever-extending lifespan, health care experts have lamented that atherosclerotic disease and the high costs of associated care have become the scourge of developed nations. Atherosclerosis underlies most vascular disease and leads to illnesses that reflect involvement of the coronary, cerebrovascular and peripheral arterial beds; dyslipidaemia is a critical factor in this pathological process.

NATIONAL AND REGIONAL DIFFERENCES

Autopsy information from international collaborations and war casualties showed by the early 1960s that early lesions of atherosclerosis were found in adults who consumed a Western diet. Fatty streaks in the aorta were present by adolescence and fibrous plaques and calcified lesions followed in early adulthood, well in advance of signs and symptoms of clinical vascular disease. The prevalence and severity of such pathological abnormalities was markedly reduced in underdeveloped regions of the world, the Mediterranean basin and in Asia.[1]

In the two decades following World War II a large number of prospective population-based studies were initiated which delineated the role of risk factors for cardiovascular disease (CVD) in various parts of the world. These investigations surveyed healthy volunteers and included a history, physical examination, blood testing and subsequent follow-up for cardiovascular events. Studies in Framingham, Chicago and Tecumseh were representative of American efforts.[2-5] European inquiries included the Seven Countries Study pioneered by Ancel Keys, and projects such as those undertaken in British civil servants and in adult volunteers from Goteborg, Sweden and Tromso, Norway.[6-8]

These observational cohort studies showed that many factors contributed to

Table 2.1   Fat intake, cholesterol levels and coronary heart disease (CHD) mortality rates, Seven Countries Study[9]

Cohort	Total fat intake (% calories)	Serum cholesterol (median in mg/dl)	CHD mortality (per 1000/10 yr)
Greece	36	201	9
Yugoslvia	31	171	12
Italy	26	198	21
Rome	–	207	22
US Railroad	40	236	57
Finland	37	259	65
Netherlands	40	230	44

increased cardiovascular risk and that blood cholesterol levels were generally higher in coronary victims.[5] Raised blood cholesterol generally correlated with greater intake of dietary saturated fat and cholesterol. The Seven Countries Study convincingly demonstrated at its outset that a high fat intake was positively related to levels of blood cholesterol (Table 2.1).[9] The regional diets responsible for these blood levels typically included a high intake of red meat, eggs and dairy products, especially at northern latitudes.

Important case–control studies were also undertaken at that time. In one investigation lipids were determined in 500 male survivors of myocardial infarction, of whom approximately 8% had elevated cholesterol, 7% had elevated triglycerides, and 15% had elevations of both lipids, giving an overall proportion of 30% with abnormal lipid levels.[10]

AGE, GENDER AND RACIAL DIFFERENCES

Migrant studies that included Japanese men from Japan, Honolulu, and San Francisco aroused interest in the 1960s. The Ni-Hon-San Study investigated levels of cholesterol and triglyceride in these three regions and tested for associations with CVD. Lipid levels tended to be lowest for the Japanese men in Japan, intermediate for the Hawaiians and highest for the San Franciscans. The incidence of coronary heart disease (CHD) showed the same trends, and the authors concluded that cholesterol and triglycerides were important determinants of cardiovascular risk. As the lipid and cardiovascular trends were evident among men who were of the same race, the differences in vascular risk were attributed to regional variations in dietary intake, especially consumption of fat and cholesterol.[11] Similar trends were not observed in another migrant study where vascular disease risk and cholesterol levels were uniformly high in all areas studied. In this instance, cholesterol levels were compared in three Irish cohorts – those born and living in Ireland, those born in Ireland who migrated to Boston, and those born in Boston to Irish immigrants. No regional differences in cholesterol levels or deaths from CHD were observed, possibly reflecting much smaller dietary differences between the Irish cohorts than those seen in the Ni-Hon-San Study.[12]

Population data from large observational studies and national surveys noted important differences in cholesterol levels according to age, gender and race. Comprehensive lipid screening was undertaken in two large American surveys during

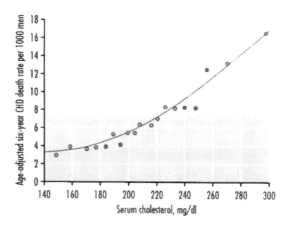

Figure 2.1 Risk of coronary heart disease (CHD) death in middle-aged men: experience of screenees for the Multiple Risk Factor Intervention Trial. Six-year follow up.[13]

the early 1970s. One survey involved screening more than 350 000 middle-aged men for the Multiple Risk Factor Intervention Trial.[13] Total cholesterol levels were strongly associated with risk of CVD death during follow-up, and the relation between cholesterol and CVD was curvilinear (Figure 2.1). At relatively low cholesterol levels in the 160 mg/dl (4.1 mmol/L) range there was little association between cholesterol and risk of cardiovascular death. Between 160 and 240 mg/dl (4.1–6.2 mmol/L) the total cholesterol to CVD death relation was strong and graded. At a cholesterol level greater than 240 mg/dl (6.2 mmol/L) the relation between cholesterol level and risk of CVD death was even stronger, reflecting a greatly increased risk. Similar data were reported in the 25-year mortality experience of the Seven Countries Study. The authors investigated the data according to lipid levels for each region (Figure 2.2).[14] The association between total cholesterol and CVD death was strongest in the American and Finnish men, intermediate for most of the European centres, and lowest for the Japanese and rural Greek participants. The authors showed that cholesterol levels at each study site were related in a linear fashion to CHD mortality. The relative increase in CHD mortality rates with a given cholesterol increase was the same. However, they also concluded that there were substantial differences in absolute risk for CHD death at any given cholesterol level, indicating that other factors were important determinants of CHD risk.

Until the late 1960s total cholesterol and triglyceride measurements in the plasma were the key determinations available for population surveys. Ultracentrifugation made it possible to separate the lipoprotein particles and some projects measured the concentration of lipids in the various particles. One of the early surveys was the Lipid Research Clinics (LRC) Program, undertaken in the 1970s. This project included analyses of total cholesterol, high density lipoprotein (HDL) cholesterol, low density lipoprotein (LDL) cholesterol, and triglycerides in a large population sample of adult Americans.[15]

The LRC survey showed that total cholesterol increased with age in both sexes up to late middle-age and declined moderately in the elderly. This comprehensive effort drew attention to the fact that the concentration of total cholesterol levels and

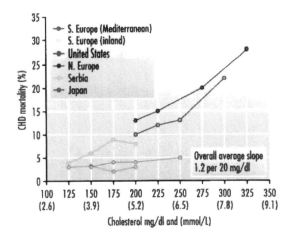

Figure 2.2 Twenty-five-year coronary heart disease (CHD) mortality risk according to baseline cholesterol level. Experience of 12 467 men participating in the Seven Countries Study. Data for each locale are shown in quartiles.[14]

its constituent particles varied with age. Although the mean cholesterol was relatively low in adolescents and only 10% of teenagers had a cholesterol >200 mg/dl (5.2 mmol/L),[16] levels generally increased between the ages of 20 and 50 years. Total cholesterol levels were relatively similar in men and women between 20 and 50 years of age, but women had higher HDL cholesterol levels at almost all ages after puberty. The typical HDL cholesterol was approximately 55 mg/dl (1.42 mmol/L) in boys and girls prior to adolescence, and 55 mg/dl (1.42 mmol/L) in women and 45 mg/dl (1.16 mmol/L) in men. After the menopause, LDL cholesterol levels increased in women and total cholesterol levels in older women typically exceeded those observed for men.[17] Total cholesterol levels were similar in Caucasian and Black population samples in the USA, but HDL cholesterol levels were generally higher in Black men.[18]

Higher levels of HDL cholesterol in women were a consistent finding in population surveys. Greater concentrations of HDL cholesterol appeared to provide protection against CVD and a reverse cholesterol transport pathway was postulated. These results offered a partial explanation for why women tended to experience lower CVD rates throughout much of their life.

A protective effect of HDL particles remained evident for men and women when total cholesterol levels were taken into account (Figure 2.3). Framingham and other investigators noted that both total and HDL cholesterol were important determinants of heart disease risk. The adverse impact of low HDL cholesterol persisted at total cholesterol levels below 200 mg/dl (5.2 mmol/L), and approximately 25% of heart attacks occurred at relatively low total cholesterol levels. Similar findings for low total cholesterol and low HDL-cholesterol were observed for both men and women.[19]

Population trend data for levels of total and HDL cholesterol are available for the USA over the past two decades. These investigations utilized precise and accurate laboratory methods and ensured that the changes were due to population differ-

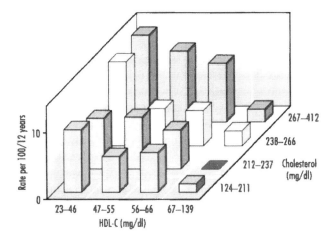

Figure 2.3 Twelve-year risk of myocardial infarction in middle-aged women according to baseline total and high density lipoprotein cholesterol (HDL-C). Framingham Heart Study experience.[19]

ences, not to variations in analytic techniques. Over this interval total cholesterol has declined modestly, but there has been little change in mean levels of HDL cholesterol on a national scale.[20] Cholesterol testing, treatment and efficacy of cholesterol lowering have also changed greatly over the past two decades and contributed to lowering of cholesterol and LDL thresholds that are targeted for life-style and pharmacological interventions, especially in the USA.[21,22]

TYPE OF RISK

Definitions of dyslipidaemia resulted from the Lipid Research Clinics Program, and it was suggested that percentile estimates should replace the traditional approach to dyslipidaemia. Scientists and public health officials agreed that a blood cholesterol >300 mg/dl (7.8 mmol/L) was elevated, but such levels were uncommon, and were not responsible for many of the cardiovascular events. Cholesterol levels >240 mg/dl (6.2 mmol/L) were noted to occur in approximately 25% of adult Americans. In the Framingham experience a cholesterol level >240 mg/dl (6.2 mmol/L) accounted for approximately 34% of the CHD events in men and 48% in women.[23] This interpretation is analogous to that for high blood pressure, where it had been noted that borderline elevations in arterial pressure often went unnoticed or untreated but contributed greatly to the population burden of disease.

Physicians have been accustomed to interpreting relative risk or relative odds – terms that express the risk of disease in a group according to a risk exposure. However, relative risk does not take into account the frequency of the exposure. Very common exposures might increase risk only mildly or moderately, but exert a dramatic effect on the overall burden of disease. An example of this phenomenon is shown in Table 2.2 for a variety of lipid disorders and lipoprotein cholesterol levels. The first column represents the prevalence of a condition, the second column shows the relative risk for CHD associated with the finding, and the third column is the population attributable risk (PAR) percentage.[24] The PAR represents a relative risk that is weighted by the prevalence of the condition and hence represents the impact of that condition on the occurrence of disease in the population. For instance, familial hypercholesterolaemia is rare and found in only 1 in 500 individuals. The relative risk for CHD is quite high, but the PAR indicates the condition is responsible for approximately only 6% of coronary disease cases. On the other hand, an LDL level >130 mg/dl (3.4 mmol/L) occurs in about two-thirds of the population and is responsible for about 18% of coronary events. Finally, data for the apolipoprotein ε4 allele are shown. This genetic marker, which occurs in about 24% of the population, appears to exert a modest increase in the relative risk for CHD and helps to account for approximately 11% of the CHD events, an impact that is similar to having an LDL cholesterol level >160 mg/dl (4.1 mmol/L).[24]

In the past, traditional risk assessment has emphasized the relative rather than the absolute risk of disease. For instance, if the absolute risk of CHD in a 35-year-old man were 2% over 10 years, and this estimate was compared with a 1% estimate over 10 years for a man the same age with very low levels of cholesterol and blood pressure, the relative odds for these persons would be estimated by the ratio of 2% to 1%, or 2:1. A similar relative odds might be obtained for a 50-year-old man with a 20% risk over 10 years compared with another man the same age with lower levels of risk factors who was estimated to have a 10% risk over 10 years. In this instance the relative odds would be the ratio of 20% to 10%, or 2:1, as in the earlier case. Relative risk estimates do not tell the complete story, however, as neither the prevalence of the condition nor its absolute risk are considered. Public health officials would be more eager to intervene in a man with a 20% absolute risk for an event than in an individual who had a 2% absolute risk. The frequency of such a risk profile is also an issue, since it is easier to develop cardiac prevention strategies when a sizeable proportion of the population are candidates, their absolute risk is high, and therapy can reduce the relative risk of a cardiovascular event.

The impact of interventions can also be estimated and some illustrations are informative. For example, if the absolute risk of a coronary disease event were 20% over the next 5 years, it is feasible that lipid-lowering therapy could reduce the absolute risk to 16%. This situation might be typical of a lipid-regulating intervention trial in persons with known CHD, that is, secondary prevention. In a second scenario the absolute risk is 10% over the next 5 years and lipid lowering reduces

Table 2.2 Prevalence of lipid risk factors, relative odds and population attributable risk percentage for coronary heart disease

Factor	Prevalence	Relative odds for CHD	PAR for CHD (%)
Familial hypercholesterolaemia	1 in 500	35	6.4
ε4 allele	24%	1.53	11
HDL <35 mg/dl	23%	2.39	24
LDL <130 mg/dl	67%	1.34	18
HDL <160 mg/dl	30%	1.41	11

CHD, coronary heart disease; PAR, population attributable risk; HDL, high density lipoprotein; LDL, low density lipoprotein.

absolute risk to 8% over the follow-up interval. This situation might represent the case of a lipid intervention for the primary prevention of CHD. How can we summarize and interpret these results?

As seen in Table 2.3, the impact of treatment on relative risk is the same for each of the groups mentioned above. On the other hand, the number needed to treat – a public health statistic that estimates the number of persons needed to treat in order to prevent a single event – provides a different perspective. The number needed to treat is much lower for the group where the absolute risk on placebo was expected to be 20% over the follow-up interval. These concepts provide the rationale of why secondary prevention is so effective and important to patients, clinicians and the population in general.

Lipid therapy has been shown to be very effective and in the recently completed lipid lowering trials the number needed to treat to prevent an event has ranged from 7–20 for secondary prevention and 40–60 for primary prevention.[25-28] Cost analyses complement these studies and show that an overall $10400 (men) and $16800 (women) per life-year were saved in direct costs for participants in the Scandinavian Simvastatin Survival Study; the extent of the savings depended on age, gender and baseline cholesterol before starting therapy. Among younger participants there was even a cost saving when both direct and indirect costs were considered in the analyses.[29]

TRENDS IN CORONARY HEART DISEASE

Death from CHD has generally decreased since the late 1960s in the USA, and a similar decline has been experienced in Canada, Australia and New Zealand. The amount of the decline has varied greatly across the regions, but a decrease of more than 30% has been typical. No single factor has been considered responsible for the decline in CHD death, and hypertension control, hospital care and treatment of persons with known heart disease are important determinants.[30,31] The overall new event rate for CHD has not decreased as dramatically, and it has been noted that myocardial infarction rates have decreased only modestly in the USA since the late 1960s.

Although CHD mortality rates have been improving or remaining stable in several regions, the rates have increased dramatically in a few, especially Eastern Europe and developing countries of the world. Reports from the late 1990s put CHD as the leading cause of death in adults[32] and projections for the interval 2000–25 list heart disease as the leading cause of disability throughout the world.[33]

Table 2.3   Expressing effects of treatment on risk

Absolute risk on placebo	Absolute risk on treatment	Relative risk reduction	Number needed to treat
20%	16%	$4/20 = 20\%$	$100/(10-16) = 25$
10%	8%	$2/10 = 20\%$	$100/(10-8) = 50$

REFERENCES

1. Eggen DA, Strong JP, McGill HCJ. Calcification in the abdominal aorta: relationship to race, sex, and coronary atherosclerosis. Arch Pathol 1964; 78:575–83.
2. Butler WJ, Ostrander LDJ, Carman WJ et al. Mortality from coronary heart disease in the Tecumseh Study: long-term effect of diabetes mellitus, glucose tolerance and other risk factors. Am J Epidemiol 1985; 121:541–7.
3. Dyer AR, Stamler J, Paul O et al. Serum cholesterol and risk of death from cancer and other causes in three Chicago epidemiological studies. J Chronic Dis 1981; 34:249.
4. Dawber TR, Meadors GF, Moore FE, Jr. Epidemiological approaches to heart disease: the Framingham Study. Am J Public Health 1951; 41:279–86.
5. Keys A. Coronary heart disease in seven countries. Circulation 1970; 41(Suppl 1):1–199.
6. Keys A, Menotti A, Aravanis C. The Seven Countries Study: 2289 deaths in 15 years. Prevent Med 1984; 13:141–54.
7. Fager G, Wiklund O, Olofsson S-O et al. Multivariate analysis of apolipoproteins and risk factors in relation to acute myocardial infarction. Arteriosclerosis 1981; 1:273–7.
8. Miller NE, Forde OH, Thelle DS et al. The Tromso Heart Study. High-density lipoprotein and coronary heart disease: a prospective case–control study. Lancet 1977; 1:965–70.
9. Keys A. The Seven Countries Study: a multivariate analysis of death and coronary heart disease, 1st edn. Cambridge: Harvard Press, 1980.
10. Goldstein JL, Hazzard WR, Schrott HG et al. Hyperlipidemia in coronary heart disease I. Lipid levels in 500 survivors of myocardial infarction. J Clin Invest 1973; 52:1533–43.
11. Kagan A, Harris BR, Winkelstein W, Jr. Epidemiologic studies of coronary disease and stroke in Japanese men living in Japan, Hawaii and California: Demographic, physical, dietary and biochemical characteristics. J Chronic Dis 1974; 27:345–64.
12. Kushi LH, Lew RA, Stare FJ et al. Diet and 20-year mortality from coronary heart disease. The Ireland–Boston Diet–Heart Study. N Engl J Med 1985; 312:811–18.
13. Neaton JD, Blackburn H, Jacobs D et al. Serum cholesterol level and mortality findings for men screened in the Multiple Risk Factor Intervention Trial. Multiple Risk Factor Intervention Trial Research Group. Arch Intern Med 1992; 152:1490–500.
14. Verschuren WM, Jacobs DR, Bloemberg BP et al. Serum total cholesterol and long-term coronary heart disease mortality in different cultures. Twenty-five-year follow-up of the Seven Countries Study. J Am Med Assoc 1995; 274:131–6.
15. Heiss G, Tamir I, Davis CE et al. Lipoprotein–cholesterol distributions in selected North American populations: the Lipid Research Clinics Program Prevalence Study. Circulation 1980; 61:302–15.
16. Glueck CJ, Stein EA. Treatment and management of hyperlipoproteinemia in childhood. In: Levy R, Rifkind B, Dennis B, Ernst N, eds. Nutrition, lipids, and coronary heart disease. New York: Raven Press, 1979:285–307.
17. Rifkind BM, Segal P. Lipid Research Clinics Program reference values for hyperlipidemia and hypolipidemia. J Am Med Assoc 1983; 250:1869–72.
18. Glueck CJ, Gartside P, Laskarzewski PM et al. High-density lipoprotein cholesterol in blacks and whites: potential ramifications for coronary heart disease. Am Heart J 1984; 108:815–26.
19. Abbott RD, Wilson PW, Kannel WB et al. High density lipoprotein cholesterol, total cholesterol screening, and myocardial infarction. The Framingham Study. Arteriosclerosis 1988; 8:207–11.
20. Sempos C, Fulwood R, Haines C et al. The prevalence of high blood cholesterol levels among adults in the United States. J Am Med Assoc 1989; 262:45–52.
21. Smith SC, Jr, Jackson R, Pearson TA et al. Principles for national and regional guidelines on cardiovascular disease prevention: a scientific statement from the World Heart and Stroke Forum. Circulation 2004; 109:3112–21.
22. Grundy SM, Cleeman JI, Merz CN et al. Implications of recent clinical trials for the

National Cholesterol Education Program Adult Treatment Panel III guidelines. Circulation 2004; 110:227–39.

23. Wilson PW, D'Agostino RB, Levy D et al. Prediction of coronary heart disease using risk factor categories. Circulation 1998; 97:1837–47.

24. Wilson PW, Myers RH, Larson MG et al. Apolipoprotein E alleles, dyslipidemia, and coronary heart disease. The Framingham Offspring Study. J Am Med Assoc 1994; 272:1666–71.

25. Downs JR, Clearfield M, Weis S et al. Primary prevention of acute coronary events with lovastatin in men and women with average cholesterol levels: results of AFCAPS/TexCAPS. J Am Med Assoc 1998; 279:1615–22.

26. Sacks FM, Pfeffer MA, Moye LA et al. The effect of pravastatin on coronary events after myocardial infarction in patients with average cholesterol levels. Cholesterol and Recurrent Events Trial investigators. N Engl J Med 1996; 335: 1001–9.

27. The 4S Group. Randomised trial of cholesterol lowering in 4444 patients with coronary heart disease: the Scandinavian Simvastatin Survival Study (4S). Lancet 1994; 344:1383–9.

28. The Long-Term Intervention with Pravastatin in Ischaemic Disease (LIPID) Study Group. Prevention of cardiovascular events and death with pravastatin in patients with coronary heart disease and a broad range of initial cholesterol levels. N Engl J Med 1998; 339:1349–57.

29. Johannesson M, Jonsson B, Kjekshus J et al. Cost effectiveness of simvastatin treatment to lower cholesterol levels in patients with coronary heart disease. Scandinavian Simvastatin Survival Study Group. N Engl J Med 1997; 336:332–6.

30. Kannel WB, Thom TJ. Implications of the recent decline in cardiovascular mortality. Cardiovasc Med 1979; 4:983–97.

31. Kannel WB. Blood pressure as a cardiovascular risk factor: prevention and treatment. J Am Med Assoc 1996; 275:1571–6.

32. Murray CJ, Lopez AD. Mortality by cause for eight regions of the world: Global Burden of Disease Study. Lancet 1997; 349:1269–76.

33. Murray CJ, Lopez AD. Alternative projections of mortality and disability by cause 1990–2020: Global Burden of Disease Study. Lancet 1997; 349:1498–504.

3

Dietary and lifestyle factors in dyslipidaemia

Introduction • Determinants of LDL cholesterol • Types of fats • Determinants of HDL cholesterol • Diabetes mellitus • Dietary interventions and cholesterol change • Alcohol and coffee • Specific nutrients

INTRODUCTION

Total cholesterol increases gradually during adult life; it generally peaks between ages 50 and 65 years, and then declines.[1] Throughout adulthood there are important changes in the distribution of total cholesterol in the plasma. The three main carriers are low density lipoprotein (LDL), high density lipoprotein (HDL), and very low density lipoprotein (VLDL). Most research has concentrated on the cholesterol concentration within each of these particle groups. Population estimates of heritability have ranged from 40% to 60% for middle-aged persons. Shared household influences are thought to be minor and add only a few per cent, leaving environmental effects to account for most of the differences in cholesterol among adults.[2] Approximately 70% of the total cholesterol is in LDL particles, 20% is in HDL particles, and only 10% is in VLDL particles. The greatest attention has been directed toward the determinants of LDL and HDL cholesterol.

DETERMINANTS OF LDL CHOLESTEROL

Dietary fat and cholesterol intake are the key environmental determinants of blood cholesterol level (Table 3.1), although other factors have an effect. Classic experiments by Hegsted and Keys in the 1950s and 1960s led to the development of metabolic ward equations that could estimate the change in cholesterol level according to changes in dietary intake of fat and cholesterol. Both Hegsted et al[3] and Keys et al[4] showed that greater saturated fat and dietary cholesterol intake tend to increase blood cholesterol (Table 3.2). On the other hand, intake of polyunsaturated fat lowers blood cholesterol levels. The magnitude of the adverse effect of saturated fat is greater than the favourable effect of polyunsaturated fat.

Some food groups contribute greatly to saturated fat and cholesterol intake. Saturated fat is generally solid at room temperature; a variety of baked goods, including cakes and biscuits, are important sources, as well as dairy products and red meat. National dietary surveys have periodically assessed the nutritional status of US residents and recent analyses have compared the intakes of cholesterol and fat from 1971 to 1991 over the course of three National Health and Nutrition Examination Surveys (NHANES).[5] Dietary fat, saturated fat, dietary cholesterol, and serum

Table 3.1 Equations to estimate change in mean serum cholesterol according to dietary fats and cholesterol

Author	Equation
Hegsted et al[3]	ΔCholesterol (mg/dl) = 2.1ΔS − 1.65ΔP + 0.0677ΔC mg/day − 0.53
Keys et al[4]	ΔCholesterol (mg/dl) = 2.7ΔS − 1.35ΔP + 1.5ΔC$^{1/2}$ mg/1000 kcal-day

For dietary components saturated fat percent of total energy intake (S), polyunsaturated fat percent of total energy intake (P), and cholesterol (C).

Table 3.2 Determinants of LDL cholesterol

Increased level	Decreased level
Greater dietary fat intake	Less dietary fat intake
Greater dietary cholesterol intake	Less dietary cholesterol intake
	Exogenous oestrogens

cholesterol all declined over the study interval. The decline in dietary cholesterol was dramatic, falling from 355 mg/day in 1972 to 318 mg/day in 1978 and reaching 291 mg/day in 1990. The median cholesterol level for all adults fell in parallel fashion from 213 mg/dl (5.5 mmol/L) in 1978 to 205 mg/dl (5.3 mmol/L) in 1990. Favourable serum cholesterol changes were observed in Whites and Blacks, both men and women. Most of the 20-year decline in total serum cholesterol was in the LDL cholesterol (LDL-C) fraction (average change −8 mg/dl or −0.21 mmol/L), and a minimal increase in HDL-C was also observed (average change −1 mg/dl or −0.03 mmol/L). Using Hegsted and Keys' equations, the authors of the NHANES dietary trends project showed that the US changes in blood cholesterol levels of US residents were predictable from the alterations that had occurred in dietary intake.[5] Between 1970 and 1990 the consumption of whole milk decreased, non-fat dairy products increased and red meat increased. The types of dietary fat are important in the determination of lipid levels and cardiovascular risk; the most recent data suggest that replacing saturated fat with unsaturated fat is a very important means of lowering risk of atherosclerotic disease.[6]

Favourable trends in blood cholesterol levels have also been observed in Finland over the past two decades. In 1972 the average cholesterol level was high (6.78 mmol/L, men; 6.72 mmol/L, women) and dropped by an average of 13% in men and 18% in women over the next 20 years. These nationwide changes, coupled with a decrease in cigarette smoking and the average blood pressure in Finland, predicted a decrease in coronary heart disease (CHD) mortality rate of 44% in men and 49% in women. In fact, the observed decline in CHD death was 55% for men and 68% for women.[7] However, not all regional changes in cholesterol levels have been favourable. Follow-up studies in Japan from the 1950s to late 1980s reported large increases in the average total cholesterol levels for adult men and women. A survey completed in the 1980s reported that the average cholesterol level rose from 157 to 179 mg/dl (4.1 to 4.6 mmol/L) in men and from 153 to 192 mg/dl (4.0 to

5.0 mmol/L) in women. Changes in average cholesterol levels were greater in urbanized regions.[8,9] The Japanese scientists noted significant changes in nutrient intake, the consumption of animal fat doubling from 4.5% of daily calories in 1969 to 9.6% in the 1980s.[9]

TYPES OF FATS

Trans isomers of fatty acids, formed by the partial hydrogenation of vegetable oils to produce margarine and vegetable shortening, have been shown to affect unfavourably the ratio of LDL-C to HDL-C and adversely influence CHD risk in large population samples.[10] Recent food labelling in the USA now identifies this type of fat in foods to alert consumers that partially hydrogenated vegetable oils act similarly to saturated fats to increase CHD risk. Grains and fish contain ω-3 polyunsaturated fatty acids, and several studies suggest they exert favourable effects on atherosclerotic risk. These unsaturated fats occur naturally and greater intake is often associated with lower levels of VLDL-C. The key ingredients are α-linolenic, eicosapentaenoic acid (EPA), and docosahexaenoic acid (DHA). Deep-water fish are especially good sources of the ω-3 fatty acids EPA and DHA. Greater intake of fish, but not necessarily fish oil supplements, has been associated with lower risk of cardiovascular disease.

The healthy effects of ω-3 fish oils are thought to be partly attributable to changes in lipids and haemostatic function.[11,12] A review of the clinical trials that used fish oil products as dietary supplements concluded that total cholesterol changed little, LDL-C increased by 5–10%, HDL-C edged upwards by 1–3% and triglycerides decreased by 25–30%. Therapy with high doses of these supplements is generally reserved for selected patients with elevated triglycerides and VLDL-C that are refractory to conventional diet and pharmacotherapy.

DETERMINANTS OF HDL CHOLESTEROL

The key factors associated with increased and decreased HDL levels are listed in Table 3.3. Weight and weight gain are key determinants. Greater weight is an important determinant of lipoprotein cholesterol levels in adulthood, as shown in Figure 3.1, which was taken from NHANES data obtained in the USA.[13] In addition, modest changes in body mass index can cause adverse effects on all of the lipid fractions. Among Framingham Heart Study participants aged 20–49 years at baseline, weight gain was associated with reductions in HDL-C and increases in total, LDL-C, and VLDL-C over 8 years of follow-up.[14] Cigarette smoking is also associated with lower HDL-C levels, and smoking cessation has been shown to lead to an increase in HDL-C levels and reduction in CHD risk for individuals and for the population at large, as recently reported for England and Wales from 1981 to 2000.[15]

Physical activity is another key determinant of HDL-C levels. Data from Stanford researchers showed that a physical activity regimen of jogging 10 miles (16 km) a week for 10 months was associated with approximately a 10% increase in HDL-C levels.[16] Weight loss interventions with exercise and diet showed that both interventions were important and that a 1-year weight loss of 5 kg in 30–59-year-old men was typically associated with an increase in HDL-C of 0.14 mmol/L. Plasma HDL-C increased significantly more in the men who exercised and dieted than in the men who only dieted. Among women, HDL-C levels remained about the same in those

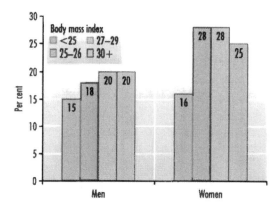

Figure 3.1   Age-adjusted prevalence of elevated cholesterol (>240 mg/dl, 6.2 mmol/L) in US National Health and Nutrition Examination Survey III according to categories of body mass index (from Expert Panel on Overweight and Obesity).[13]

Table 3.3   Determinants of HDL cholesterol

Increased level	Decreased level
Leanness	Obesity
Oestrogen	Androgens
Alcohol intake	Cigarette smoking
Exercise	Inactivity
Genetic	Genetic

who exercised and dieted and were higher in women who only dieted, but not higher than controls. The authors concluded that regular exercise in overweight men and women enhanced the improvement in lipids that results from the adoption of a low saturated fat, low cholesterol diet.[17] Studies from observational studies have shown that regular physical activity has been consistently associated with greater levels of HDL-C in men and women. As seen in the Framingham Study, mean levels of HDL-C were 42 mg/dl (1.09 mmol/L) in men who performed little aerobic activity (<1 h/week) and 47.8 mg/dl (1.24 mmol/L) in their counterparts who were aerobically active (>1 h/week). Corresponding mean levels for women were 53.5 mg/dl (1.38 mmol/L) for those who were inactive and 61.1 mg/dl (1.58 mmol/L) for those who were aerobically active (Figure 3.2).[18]

DIABETES MELLITUS

Diabetes mellitus increases risk of CHD approximately twofold in younger men and threefold in younger women. Part of this increased risk is attributable to differences in lipoprotein cholesterol levels: HDL-C levels are lower, VLDL-C and triglyceride levels are higher, but usually little difference in total cholesterol or LDL-C levels is

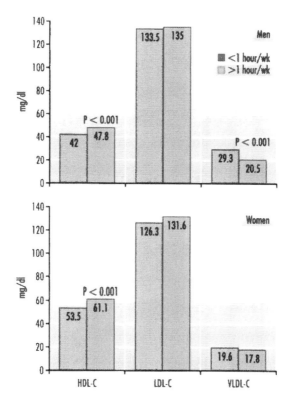

Figure 3.2 Reported usual physical activity and mean lipid levels in Framingham Heart Study Offspring 20–59 years of age (adapted from Dannenberg).[18]

observed. The impact of diabetes on lipid levels appears to be greater in women than in men. Pronounced differences in lipids in diabetic patients are seen if comparisons are made for extreme lipid values in studies which go beyond simply reporting the impact of the condition on mean levels of lipoprotein cholesterol (Figure 3.3).[19]

DIETARY INTERVENTIONS AND CHOLESTEROL CHANGE

Throughout the 1960s a large number of dietary intervention studies were undertaken in an effort to prevent initial or recurrent coronary artery disease. These investigations preceded the era of potent lipid medications that began in the 1980s. Many of the dietary interventions had little effect on the blood cholesterol level but several were effective in reducing blood cholesterol by 10–15% and decreasing CHD risk by 20–30%.[20] A similar effect has been observed for the less potent cholesterol lowering medications when total cholesterol is reduced in the 10–20% range compared to baseline.

The usual American diet contains approximately 35–38% calories as fat, and US experts have recommended that all adults should consume no more than 30% of

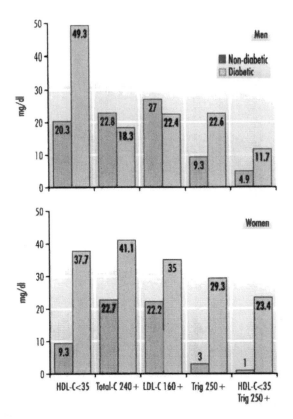

Figure 3.3   Diabetes mellitus and mean lipid levels in Framingham Heart Study Offspring (adapted from Siegel).[19]

their calories as fat, following a step 1 diet (Figure 3.4). It has been estimated that such goals are achievable, would reduce blood cholesterol approximately 10%, and might decrease CHD events by 20% over a 5-year period for middle-aged adults.[21] Persons with mildly elevated cholesterol should follow the step 1 diet, the major difference between the latter and their usual diet being the limitation of saturated fat intake.

More aggressive cholesterol lowering often necessitates use of lipid medications, but diet continues to have an important role for those patients. Favourable effects on cardiovascular risk were obtained for a low fat, low cholesterol diet in persons who were also on statin therapy.[20-25] If the step 1 diet does not achieve the target cholesterol level, it is possible to try more aggressive dietary programmes. The step 2 diet (26% total fat, 4% saturated fat, 45 mg cholesterol/1000 kcal) is often the next choice. Many diets have been presented to the public as cardioprotective, and Figure 3.4 shows that the nutrient content of many of these diets are very similar.

In order to follow this regimen and ensure adequate intake of certain nutrients and essential fatty acids nutritional counselling is recommended. Cholesterol levels declined for persons who followed step 2 diet for 24 weeks after a lead-in period on

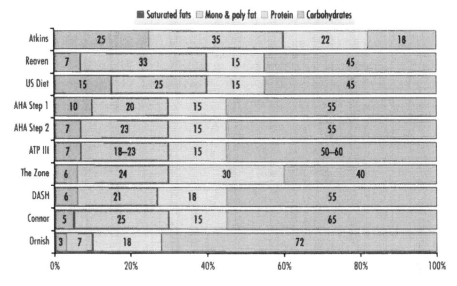

Figure 3.4 Estimated nutrient intake in various diets. Mono & poly fat = fat containing mono- and polyunsaturated fatty acids. Taken from a variety of sources, including Ornish,[22] Lichtenstein,[23] Atkins,[24] Appel,[26] and Expert Panel ATP III.[25] DASH, Dietary Approaches to Stop Hypertension (study).

the usual American diet (35% calories as total fat, 14% saturated fat, 147 mg cholesterol/1000 kcal). The LDL-C level declined 18% and HDL-C fell 15% in persons on this diet who had elevated cholesterol levels at the start of the trial.

There is variability in blood cholesterol response to dietary reduction in fat and cholesterol. One investigation found a gene–environment interaction; men with the apolipoprotein E3/4 or E4/4 genotype experiencing a significantly greater decrease in LDL-C (−24%) with the step 2 diet than men with the E3/3 genotype (−18%). The authors concluded that almost half of the variability in the plasma LDL-C response could be accounted for by baseline LDL concentrations and age in men.

Estimates for several dietary programmes are shown in Figure 3.4. Diets that restrict fat and calories more aggressively than the US step 2 diet are difficult to follow for extended periods, although the Ornish diet is an example of a very restrictive diet that appears to be effective. Participants in that programme experienced improvements in coronary angiography after 1 year, better myocardial perfusion after 5 years, and a reduced need for coronary revascularization.[22,27,28]

ALCOHOL AND COFFEE

Greater intake of alcohol is associated with higher levels of HDL cholesterol levels in men and women, although consumption of more than two alcoholic beverages per day is uncommon in women.[29] Risk of CHD is also associated with greater intake of alcohol and it does not appear that the type of alcoholic beverage consumed exerts a significant effect.[30] Beyond two drinks a day in men, or one drink a day in women, there is an increased risk in non-cardiovascular causes of death, including trauma, cancer, and liver disease.[31] Higher levels of blood cholesterol have been related to greater intake of boiled coffee over a 1-month interval.[32] Consumption of boiled coffee may help to explain higher cholesterol levels and greater rates of CHD in Norway in the past. A switch from boiled coffee to filtered coffee, greater intake of antioxidants, and lower cholesterol levels has occurred in Norway since 1960. These trends in coffee and antioxidant intake may help to explain the 30% decline in CHD risk that has been observed there in the intervening period.[33]

SPECIFIC NUTRIENTS

Several individual nutrients may have effects on blood cholesterol levels. This section will consider a few of them, but many other candidates exist. Oats are a rich source of a water-soluble fibre β-glucan and clinical trials have been conducted with oatmeal and oat bran in the diet. Consumption of both oat products was associated with reductions in LDL-C over 6 weeks. The oat products led to approximately 10–15% lowering in LDL-C, the effects depended on the dose, and oat bran resulted in more pronounced LDL-C lowering than similar amounts of oatmeal.[34] Exponents of greater fibre intake note that we are eating much less fibre than recommended and increased consumption should lead to improvements in cholesterol, coronary disease risk, glucose control, and gastrointestinal diseases.[35] Other sources of fibre may have similar effects, and psyllium products that are often used to avoid constipation may reduce cholesterol levels by a few per cent.[36]

Consumption of nuts more than four times a week was associated with a 50% lower risk of CHD death among persons in the California Seventh Day Adventist Study. The authors suggested that a favourable fatty acid profile of many nuts may be responsible for the effects, but it is likely that other healthy habits contributed.[37] Soy protein, a common grain product in Asian diets, has become a more popular nutrient in other regions. In clinical trials over a 1-month period, a tofu-based diet was associated with lower levels of total cholesterol (-0.23 mmol/L), HDL cholesterol (-0.08 mmol/L) and triglycerides (-0.15 mmol/L) compared with lean meat.[38] Increased intake of soy protein products may lead to reduced consumption of foods that are high in saturated fat and cholesterol and this substitution may contribute to blood cholesterol lowering.[39]

REFERENCES

1. Greenland P, Knoll MD, Stamler J et al. Major risk factors as antecedents of fatal and non-fatal coronary heart disease events. J Am Med Assoc 2003; 290:891–7.
2. Sing CF, Moll PP. Genetics of variability of CHD risk. Int J Epidemiol 1989; 18(Suppl 1): S183–S95.
3. Hegsted DM, McGandy RB, Myers ML, Stare FJ. Quantitative effects of dietary fat on serum cholesterol in man. Am J Clin Nutr 1965; 17:281–95.
4. Keys A, Anderson JT, Grande F. Serum cholesterol response to changes in the diet. II. The effect of cholesterol in the diet. Metabolism 1965; 14:749–65.
5. Ernst ND, Sempos CT, Briefel RR, Clark MB. Consistency between US dietary fat intake and serum total cholesterol concentrations: the National Health and Nutrition Examination Surveys. Am J Clin Nutr 1997; 66(Suppl):965S–72S.
6. Hu FB, Manson JE, Willett WC. Types of dietary fat and risk of coronary heart disease: a critical review. J Am Coll Nutr 2001; 20:5–19.
7. Vartiainen E, Puska P, Pekkanen J et al. Changes in risk factors explain changes in mortality from ischaemic heart disease in Finland. Br Med J 1994; 309:23–7.

8. Yamada M, Wong FL, Kodama K et al. Longitudinal trends in total serum cholesterol levels in a Japanese cohort, 1958–1986. J Clin Epidemiol 1997; 50:425–34.
9. Shimamoto T, Komachi Y, Inada H et al. Trends for coronary heart disease and stroke and their risk factors in Japan. Circulation 1989; 79:503–15.
10. Willett WC, Stampfer MJ, Manson JE et al. Intake of trans fatty acids and risk of coronary heart disease among women. Lancet 1993; 341:581–5.
11. Kromhout D, Basschieter EBB, de Lezenne-Contander C. The inverse relation between fish consumption and 20-year mortality from coronary heart disease. N Engl J Med 1985; 312:1205–9.
12. Knapp HR, Reilly IAG, Alessandrini P, FitzGerald GA. In vivo indexes of platelet and vascular function during fish-oil administration in patients with atherosclerosis. N Engl J Med 1986; 314:937–42.
13. Expert Panel. Clinical Guidelines on the Identification, Evaluation, and Treatment of Overweight and Obesity in Adults. Bethesda, MD: Public Health Service, National Institutes of Health, National Heart, Lung, and Blood Institute, 1998.
14. Anderson KM, Wilson PWF, Garrison RJ, Castelli WP. Longitudinal and secular trends in lipoprotein cholesterol measurements in a general population sample: The Framingham Offspring Study. Atherosclerosis 1987; 68:59–66.
15. Unal B, Critchley JA, Capewell S. Explaining the decline in coronary heart disease mortality in England and Wales between 1981 and 2000. Circulation 2004; 109:1101–7.
16. Wood PD, Haskell WL, Blair SN et al. Increased exercise level and plasma lipoprotein concentration. A one-year, randomized controlled study in sedentary, middle-aged men. Metabolism 1983; 32:31–9.
17. Wood PD, Stefanick ML, Williams PT, Haskell WL. The effects on plasma lipoproteins of a prudent weight-reducing diet, with or without exercise, in overweight men and women. N Engl J Med 1991; 325:461–6.
18. Dannenberg AL, Keller JB, Wilson PWF, Castelli WP. Leisure time physical activity in the Framingham Offspring Study. Description, seasonal variation, and risk factor correlates. Am J Epidemiol 1989; 129:76–87.
19. Siegel RD, Cupples A, Schaefer EJ, Wilson PW. Lipoproteins, apolipoproteins, and low-density lipoprotein size among diabetics in the Framingham offspring study. Metabolism 1996; 45:1267–72.
20. Castelli WP. Epidemiology of coronary heart disease: the Framingham Study. Am J Med 1984; 76:4–12.
21. Gotto AM, Jr., LaRosa JC, Hunninghake D et al. The cholesterol facts: a summary of the evidence relating dietary fats, serum cholesterol, and coronary heart disease: a joint statement by the American Heart Association and the National, Heart, Lung, and Blood Institute. Circulation 1990; 81:1721–33.
22. Ornish D, Brown SE, Scherwitz LW et al. Can lifestyle changes reverse coronary heart disease? The Lifestyle Heart Trial. Lancet 1990; 336:129–33.
23. Lichtenstein AH. Soy protein, isoflavonoids, and risk of developing coronary heart disease. Curr Atheroscl Rep 1999; 1:210–14.
24. Atkins RC. Dr Atkins' new diet revolution. New York: Avon, 1997.
25. Executive Summary of The Third Report of The National Cholesterol Education Program (NCEP) Expert Panel on Detection, Evaluation, and Treatment of High Blood Cholesterol In Adults (Adult Treatment Panel III). J Am Med Assoc 2001; 285:2486–97.
26. Appel LJ, Moore TJ, Obarzanek E et al. A clinical trial of the effects of dietary patterns on blood pressure. DASH Collaborative Research Group. N Engl J Med 1997; 336:1117–24.
27. Gould KL, Ornish D, Scherwitz L et al. Changes in myocardial perfusion abnormalities by positron emission tomography after long-term, intense risk factor modification. J Am Med Assoc 1995; 274:894–901.
28. Ornish D. Avoiding revascularization with lifestyle changes: the Multicenter Lifestyle Demonstration Project. Am J Cardiol 1998; 82:72T–6T.

29. Castelli WP, Doyle JT, Gordon T et al. Alcohol and blood lipids. The cooperative lipoprotein phenotyping study. Lancet 1977; 2:153–5.
30. Gaziano JM, Hennekens CH, Godfried SL et al. Type of alcoholic beverage and risk of myocardial infarction. Am J Cardiol 1999; 83:52–7.
31. Ellison RC. Cheers! Epidemiology 1990; 1:337–9.
32. Aro A, Tuomilehto J, Kostiainen E et al. Boiled coffee increases serum low density lipoprotein concentration. Metabolism 1987; 36:1027–30.
33. Johansson L, Drevon CA, Aa Bjorneboe GE. The Norwegian diet during the last hundred years in relation to coronary heart disease. Eur J Clin Nutr 1996; 50:277–83.
34. Davidson MH, Dugan LD, Burns JH et al. The hypocholesterolemic effects of beta-glucan in oatmeal and oat bran. A dose-controlled study. J Am Med Assoc 1991; 265:1833–9.
35. Rimm EB, Ascherio A, Giovannucci E et al. Vegetable, fruit, and cereal fiber intake and risk of coronary heart disease among men. J Am Med Assoc 1996; 275:447–51.
36. Schectman G, Hiatt J, Hartz A. Evaluation of the effectiveness of lipid-lowering therapy (bile acid sequestrants, niacin, psyllium and lovastatin) for treating hypercholesterolemia in veterans. Am J Cardiol 1993; 71:759–65.
37. Fraser GE, Sabate J, Beeson WL, Strahan TM. A possible protective effect of nut consumption on risk of coronary heart disease. The Adventist Health Study. Arch Intern Med 1992; 152:1416–24.
38. Ashton E, Ball M. Effects of soy as tofu vs meat on lipoprotein concentrations. Eur J Clin Nutr 2000; 54:14–19.
39. Lichtenstein AH. Soy protein, isoflavones and cardiovascular disease risk. J Nutr 1998; 128:1589–92.

4

Screening for dyslipidaemia

Why screen for dyslipidaemia? • What is the best screening test for dyslipidaemia? • Do we need to screen for dyslipidaemia? • Who should be screened for dyslipidaemia? • Screening for familial hypercholesterolaemia • Age considerations • Where should screening for dyslipidaemia take place? • When and how should screening for dyslipidaemia take place in primary care? • 'Positive' screening

'I keep six honest serving-men
(They taught me all I knew);
Their names are What and Why and When
And How and Where and Who'

Rudyard Kipling (1865–1936)

WHY SCREEN FOR DYSLIPIDAEMIA?

Cardiovascular disease is very common

Cardiovascular disease (CVD) has become such a global scourge that by 1990 it was clear that coronary heart disease (CHD) (with 6.3 million deaths) and cerebrovascular disease (with 4.4 million deaths) were the two leading causes of death worldwide.[1] The situation has been particularly acute in the developed societies of Western Europe and North America where the prevalence of the main manifestations of CVD has been of epidemic proportions for some decades (see Table 4.1).

Cardiovascular disease is set to become more common

A number of subtle, secular patterns are emerging in different societies around the world which look set to fuel CVD for years to come. These include:

Table 4.1 Prevalence of cardiovascular mortality: USA (2002) and UK (2003)

	CVD deaths	% total deaths	CHD deaths	Stroke deaths
USA 2002	927 448	38	494 382	162 672
UK 2003	233 000	38	113 895	65 764

Sources: Heart Disease and Stroke Statistics – 2005 American Heart Association (website), British Heart Foundation Statistics Database 2005 (website). CVD, cardiovascular disease; CHD, coronary heart disease.

- The acquisition of increased cardiovascular risk by low development cultures as they adopt the lifestyle habits of more developed ones. Reduced physical activity, smoking and a diet high in total fat (particularly saturated fat), cholesterol, sugar, salt, alcohol and unnecessary calories and low in potassium, fibre and other essential nutrients are an established recipe for atherosclerotic disease.
- The burden of ageing. In developed societies the ageing of the population will undoubtedly result in an increasing incidence of CVD, including CHD, heart failure and stroke.
- Increased socioeconomic and ethnic inequalities within cultures.
- An alarming increase in unattended risk factors in younger generations.
- The increasing prevalence of obesity, diabetes mellitus and metabolic syndrome in association with their related complications of dyslipidaemia and hypertension. The prevalence of metabolic syndrome in the USA rises to as high as 43.5% in people aged 60–69 years. The prevalence of overweight, obesity and diabetes mellitus in the USA and the UK are shown in Table 4.2.

Dyslipidaemia is a central risk factor for cardiovascular disease

In 2002, the World Health Report estimated in developed countries, that 60% of CHD and nearly 40% of ischaemic stroke are associated with cholesterol levels in excess of a theoretical maximum of 3.8 mmol/L.[2] We have seen in Chapter 2 the importance of dyslipidaemia as a risk factor for CVD and that the influence of dyslipidaemia on cardiovascular risk extends beyond total and low density lipoprotein (LDL) cholesterol such that the other lipoproteins, notably high density lipoprotein (HDL) cholesterol and triglyceride-rich lipoproteins, also contribute significantly to risk.

National initiatives promote the identification of high-risk individuals

The burden of the problem of CVD, the central role of dyslipidaemia in the various manifestations of atherosclerotic disease, and the evidence base for intervention, have led to a number of national initiatives for the prevention of cardiovascular risk. These broadly support the parallel strategies of population-based prevention and an individual, or high-risk approach, whereby individuals at high risk of CVD are identified and prioritized for treatment.[3-5] In the UK, the National Service Framework (NSF) for CHD advocates first the identification of individuals with estab-

Table 4.2 Percentages of the British and American populations who are overweight, obese or have been diagnosed with diabetes mellitus

		% overweight BMI > 25	% obese BMI > 30	% with diabetes mellitus
USA (2002)	Men	69	28	7
	Women	62	33	6
UK (2003)	Men	43	22	4
	Women	33	23	3

Sources: Heart Disease and Stroke Statistics – 2005 American Heart Association (website), British Heart Foundation Statistics Database 2005 (website). BMI, body mass index.

lished atherosclerotic disease for treatment and subsequently those at high risk who have yet to develop symptoms.[6] Identifying people at risk implies some sort of screening programme and the NSF has been criticized for limiting initial screening in asymptomatic individuals to those with the established diagnoses of diabetes and hypertension, limiting the upper age limit to 74 years and also choosing the relatively high threshold of >30% 10-year CHD risk for drug intervention.

The original meaning of the word 'screen' was a sieve. Sieves trap certain particles by their meshwork, but others slip through the holes. Sometimes the wrong particles are retained and the right ones escape. In the same way all screening programmes have false positives and false negatives, something which both health care professionals and the public often fail to understand.

To be successful, a screening programme should be managed according to a series of defined criteria, mostly derived from the work of Wilson and Jungner,[7] which relate to:

- The condition itself. (Is it important? Do we understand the natural history of the condition? Is there a latent or early symptomatic stage? Is there a detectable risk factor or disease marker?)
- The test. (Is there a suitable, acceptable, simple, safe, precise, validated test with a defined pathway for positive results?)
- The treatment. (Is treatment beneficial, evidence-based and available?)
- The screening programme. (Is it effective, acceptable, safe, cost-effective and quality assured, and are the implications understood by those being screened?)

WHAT IS THE BEST SCREENING TEST FOR DYSLIPIDAEMIA?

Within a population the relationship between blood cholesterol levels and CHD has been established beyond question by powerful databases such as from the Multiple Risk Factor Intervention Trial (MRFIT).[8] For an individual, however, knowledge of the total cholesterol level is less predictive and fails to distinguish accurately

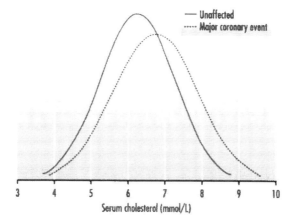

Figure 4.1 Serum cholesterol distribution in 438 men who had a major coronary event and 7252 unaffected men. Reproduced from Pocock et al,[9] with permission.

Table 4.3 Likelihood ratios for coronary heart disease of various lipid profiles, Framingham Study, Examination II

Lipid profile	Men	Women
TC	1.98 ns	2.26 ns
LDL-C	4.39	4.53
HDL-C	14.03	21.21
Triglyceride	0.51 ns	9.52
TC/HDL-C	17.11	20.41

TC, total cholesterol; LDL, low density lipoprotein; HDL, high density lipoprotein; ns, not significant.

between individuals who go on to develop CHD and those who do not. Most people who have heart attacks have average levels of cholesterol and their heart attacks are caused by the interactive influence of other risk factors as well as cholesterol (see Figure 4.1).[9] Trying to interpret the influence of total cholesterol readings on risk is analogous to trying to investigate anaemia without access to measures of red cell morphology or haematinic factors.

Data from the Framingham study show that the uncertainty associated with total cholesterol measurements can be offset by measuring the full lipoprotein profile. Likelihood ratios for various lipid profiles of CHD are shown in Table 4.3.

The ratio of total cholesterol to HDL cholesterol emerges as an efficient lipid risk predictor, which is endorsed by the recommendations of the Joint British Societies.[3] For screening purposes, a non-fasting serum cholesterol and non-fasting HDL cholesterol are adequate and will facilitate the estimation of cardiovascular risk when assessed with other cardiovascular risk factors (see Chapters 5 and 6). If dyslipidaemia is found, or if lipid-lowering therapy is being contemplated, patients should have a full fasting profile to include cholesterol, HDL cholesterol and triglycerides to define the pattern of dyslipidaemia present and enable LDL cholesterol to be calculated. Additional blood tests – fasting blood glucose, thyroid stimulating hormone (TSH) and tests of liver and renal function – can be performed at this stage to exclude secondary dyslipidaemia.

Cholesterol levels themselves are subject to a number of influences within an individual, and intra-individual differences are seen as a result of changes in diet, menstruation and pregnancy, both during and after acute illness. This biological variation can be further compounded by sampling errors and laboratory imprecision, thus emphasizing the importance of repeated testing, particularly in the diagnostic and assessment settings.

In the USA, the strategy is different and the fasting lipoprotein profile is recommended from the outset.[4] In primary prevention, total and HDL cholesterol levels are used to help define cardiovascular risk by means of a point scoring system, but thereafter treatment decisions and targets are heavily based on LDL cholesterol (see Chapters 5 and 6).

The purpose of screening for dyslipidaemia is to identify those with an increased risk of developing CVD or experiencing a further cardiovascular event. When dyslipidaemia is found, its contribution to cardiovascular risk is then assessed and the overall cardiovascular risk defined for the individual, expressed as the percentage risk of a cardiovascular event or death over a period of time. Each international guideline includes risk calculation algorithms or charts which act as decision aids and these are discussed in Chapter 6.[3-5] Risk assessment combining multiple risk factors is preferable to focusing on arbitrary thresholds of single risk factors, but practical issues remain concerning the accuracy of risk assessment and the sharing of the decisions with patients.

DO WE NEED TO SCREEN FOR DYSLIPIDAEMIA?

The Heart Protection Study showed that treatment for dyslipidaemia benefits individuals at significant risk of cardiovascular events, irrespective of their baseline cholesterol levels.[10] This led some commentators to suggest that screening for dyslipidaemia was superfluous, and that what mattered was to effect a 1 mmol/L reduction in LDL cholesterol in all at-risk individuals to achieve the outcomes predicted by the Heart Protection Study. The problems with this approach are several, not least that the lipid profile is an important determinant of cardiovascular risk in the first place. Such an approach also fails to identify subtleties of the lipoprotein profile, which might suggest more aggressive management; furthermore, genetic dyslipidaemias are missed and the attendant possibility of family screening. Finally, patients are interested in following their lipid profile results and this can be an important factor to harness in facilitating treatment persistence.

WHO SHOULD BE SCREENED FOR DYSLIPIDAEMIA?

Owing to its major role in the development of atherosclerotic CVD, screening for dyslipidaemia should ultimately be universal and available as part of cardiovascular risk assessment for all adults on a regular basis. This approach is already supported by the National Cholesterol Education Program in America, where full profile screening is recommended in all adults over 20 years every 5 years.[4] The task, however, is enormous and most authorities advise a targeted, selective approach to screening based on priority groups who, by their high-risk nature, would have most to gain by modification of their dyslipidaemic profile.

The priority groups are as follows:

1. *People with pre-existing atherosclerotic disease (CHD, stroke and transient ischaemic attack, peripheral arterial disease including erectile dysfunction) and diabetes (for 'secondary prevention')*. The significance of pre-existing disease is so strong that, ironically, the most effective screening question for defining an individual at high risk of a cardiovascular event is, 'Do you have heart disease?' The presence of diabetes, with its high risk of CVD, is now accepted as a CVD risk equivalent.
2. *People without diagnosed atherosclerotic disease whose risk of cardiovascular disease is high (for 'primary prevention')*. As thresholds for therapeutic intervention fall, more individuals become potentially eligible for treatment. People with obesity (increased body mass index or waist circumference), hypertension, and those who smoke, form potential target groups for dyslipidaemia screening, but also those with less common illnesses such as chronic renal failure or HIV infection, whose risk of CVD is also high.
3. *People with an adverse family history of CVD*. Familial dyslipidaemias are often

identified where there is a predisposition towards CVD within the family pedigree, particularly when cardiovascular events occur at an early age (<55 years for male relatives, <65 years for females).

4. *People with stigmata of dyslipidaemia.* Typically, stigmata include xanthelasma, corneal arcus and xanthomata (see Chapter 5).

SCREENING FOR FAMILIAL HYPERCHOLESTEROLAEMIA

The tragedy of undetected cases of familial hypercholesterolaemia (FH) is all too common and affected men often die from CHD before the age of 50 years. These deaths are all the more tragic because treatment is both safe and effective. In the UK, only about a quarter of cases are known and most are not diagnosed until middle age.[11] To compound the tragedy, screening is often not extended to other, asymptomatic, family members who may also be affected. Affected individuals can be identified in childhood with established guidelines for testing from the age of 2 years.[12] In the Netherlands, Kastelein's group screened all 5442 relatives of 237 people with FH and included LDL-receptor gene mutation analysis.[13] DNA testing enabled 2039 further individuals to be diagnosed with heterozygous FH and 18% of these would have been misdiagnosed by cholesterol testing alone.

In 2004, in conjunction with the cholesterol charity HEART UK, the British government initiated a pilot cascade screening programme to find the best way of identifying affected relatives with FH.

AGE CONSIDERATIONS

Although relatives of individuals with genetic dyslipidaemia may be identified from very young ages, the majority of individuals with dyslipidaemia are identified in adult life. Screening is reasonable from the age of 20 years, particularly for individuals in the priority groups. As a minimum, measuring the cholesterol in all individuals over the age of 50 years was found in one study to identify 92.8% of those at

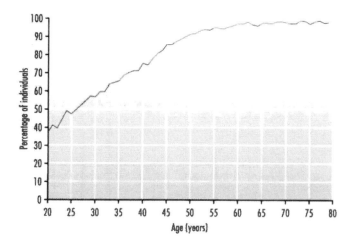

Figure 4.2 Prevalence of men and women aged 20–79 years with serum cholesterol ≥5 mmol/L in The Nord–Trondelag Health Study. Modified from Westin and Heath,[15] with permission.

15% 10-year CHD risk or more.[14] Getz has shown that in a Norwegian population, 90% of individuals have cholesterol levels of 5.0 mmol/L or more by the age of 50 years[15] (Figure 4.2).

The more difficult question is defining an upper age limit for screening for dyslipidaemia. Epidemiological studies show that the association between dyslipidaemia and CVD decreases with age, but as the burden of such disease in the elderly is so much greater; the overall risk attributable to dyslipidaemia actually increases. This means that measures to reduce cholesterol in older people are potentially highly effective. The Heart Protection Study and PROSPER recruited patients up to 80 years and 82 years, respectively and with follow-up this means that we have intervention trial data to 85 years.[10,16] In the former study, major cardiovascular events were reduced in individuals between 75 and 80 years by nearly a third, and reduced overall in the latter study by 15%.

WHERE SHOULD SCREENING FOR DYSLIPIDAEMIA TAKE PLACE?

For the most part, screening for dyslipidaemia has traditionally been undertaken in primary care, with secondary care active on an opportunistic basis. Recent developments have seen an extension of testing into the commercial arena (where pharmacists and other independent providers are active) and occupational health (within employee health checks). Wherever screening takes place, certain pathways of care should be in place including the availability of pre-test counselling and accurate testing, the ability to communicate and interpret results and to give advice on actions required. It is important that all of these actions should be underpinned by appropriate clinical governance.

Primary care remains well placed to fulfil all these expectations and provide coherent, holistic, management plans with long-term care pathways that are more likely to foster compliance with the lifestyle and pharmacological modifications required to reduce cardiovascular risk.

WHEN AND HOW SHOULD SCREENING FOR DYSLIPIDAEMIA TAKE PLACE IN PRIMARY CARE?

Screening for dyslipidaemia in primary care should be a continuous programme. Formal screening by a call and recall system is hard to co-ordinate and many do not respond to the initial invitation. Informal or opportunistic screening can take place at any primary care contact and spreading the task over years allows the possibility of tackling the large numbers involved. As 70% of patients visit their primary care physician annually, and 90–95% over a 5-year period, most of the practice can be screened. As those in social classes IV and V attend more regularly, there is opportunity to address the groups most at need. More formal opportunities for screening exist at new patient interviews, well-person checks or designated clinics for diabetes, hypertension, obesity management, smoking cessation or CVD prevention.

All forms of screening carry the potential for harm. While screening programmes may benefit populations, not all participants will benefit from participation and some will even be harmed by it. Labelling an individual as dyslipidaemic or at high cardiovascular risk creates demands for clinical monitoring and adherence to treatment as well as creating the possibility of a life lived in fear of a heart attack or stroke. In recognition of this, a policy shift is occurring, such that people participating in screening programmes do so on the basis of informed choice.[17]

Having informed choice means being given good quality and relevant information, expressed in terms that are accessible to the individual. In the context of screening for dyslipidaemia this means understanding not only the meaning and potential implications of test results, but also the concept of cardiovascular risk. The positive side of screening, when individuals have given their consent through informed choice, is improved compliance with subsequent treatment initiatives.

'POSITIVE' SCREENING

Although a major risk factor, dyslipidaemia is but one component of cardiovascular risk. Evaluating the significance of an individual's lipid profile within the context of their global cardiovascular risk demands a holistic approach and health care practitioners involved in dyslipidaemia screening need to assess a number of risk factors in order to define the level of risk and decide on a management plan. The most important factors to consider are shown in Table 4.4. The process of cardiovascular risk assessment and guidelines for the management of dyslipidaemia according to cardiovascular risk status are discussed in Chapters 5, 6 and 8.

Table 4.4   Major factors to be taken into consideration in cardiovascular risk assessment

Age
Sex
Personal or family history of cardiovascular disease
Ethnicity
Lipid profile
Blood pressure
Smoking habit
Glucose tolerance
Physical activity
Dietary habit
Alcohol consumption
Weight (body mass index or waist circumference)
Psychosocial factors and suitability for treatment
Concomitant disease and drug therapy

REFERENCES

1. Murray CJL, Lopez AD. Global burden of disease study. Lancet 1997; 349:1269–76, 1347–52 and 1436–42.
2. World Health Report 2002. Geneva: World Health Organization (WHO) website. Available at: http://www.who. int/whr/2002/en/whr02-en.pdf [July 05].
3. Wood D, Durrington P, Poulter N et al. Joint British recommendations on prevention of coronary heart disease in clinical practice. Heart 1998; 80(Suppl 2):S1–29.
4. Expert Panel on Detection, Evaluation and Treatment of High Blood Cholesterol in Adults 2001. Executive Summary of the Third Report of the National Cholesterol Education Program (NCEP) Expert Panel on Detection, Evaluation and Treatment of High Blood Cholesterol in Adults (Adult Treatment Panel III). J Am Med Assoc 2001; 285:2486–97.

5. De Backer G, Ambrosioni E, Borch-Johnsen K et al. European guidelines on cardiovascular disease prevention in clinical practice: Third Joint Task Force of European and other Societies on Cardiovascular Disease Prevention in Clinical Practice. Eur Heart J 2003; 24:1601–10.
6. Department of Health. National Service Framework for coronary heart disease. Modern standards and service models. London: Department of Health, 2000.
7. Wilson JMJ, Jungner JJ. Principles and practice of screening for disease. Geneva: World Health Organization, 1968.
8. Stamler J. Findings of the Multiple Risk Factor Intervention Trial. J Am Med Assoc 1986; 254:2823–8.
9. Pocock SJ, Shaper AG, Phillips AN. Concentrations of high density lipoprotein cholesterol, triglycerides and total cholesterol in ischaemic heart disease. Br Med J 1989; 298:998–1002.
10. Heart Protection Study Collaborative Group. MRC/BHF Heart Protection Study of cholesterol lowering with simvastatin in 20 536 high-risk individuals: a randomised placebo-controlled trial. Lancet 2002; 360:7–22.
11. Neil HAW, Hammond T, Huxley R et al. Extent of underdiagnosis of familial hypercholesterolaemia in routine practice: prospective registry study. Br Med J 2000; 321:148.
12. Neil H, Rees A, Taylor C, eds 1996. Hyperlipidaemia in childhood. London: Royal College of Physicians.
13. Umans-Eckenhausen MAW, Defesche JC, Sijbrands EJG et al. Review of first 5 years of screening for familial hypercholesterolaemia in the Netherlands. Lancet 2001; 357:165–8.
14. Wilson J, Johnston A, Robson J et al. Comparison of methods to identify individuals at increased risk of coronary disease from the general population. Br Med J 2003; 326:1436–8.
15. Getz L, Kirkengen AL, Hetlevik I et al. Ethical dilemmas arising from implementation of the European guidelines on cardiovascular disease prevention in clinical practice. Scand J Primary Health Care 2004; 22:202–8.
16. Shepherd J, Blauw GJ, Murphy MB et al. Pravastatin in elderly individuals at risk of vascular disease (PROSPER): a randomised controlled trial. Lancet 2002; 360:1623–30.
17. National Screening Committee. Second Report of the UK National Screening Committee. Departments of Health for England, Scotland, Northern Ireland and Wales, 2000. Available at: www.doh.gov. uk/nsc/pdfs/secondreport.pdf [July 05].

5

Clinical assessment of dyslipidaemia

History • Examination • Laboratory tests • Electrocardiographic abnormalities • Quantification of coronary heart disease risk • Non-invasive indices of pre-clinical vascular disease

HISTORY

Dyslipidaemic patients are usually detected on screening rather than presenting with symptoms or signs directly attributable to their dyslipidaemia. However, the fact that they are often asymptomatic at the time of presentation does not obviate the need to take a history and examine them.

When taking the current history, enquiries should be made regarding the existence of any symptoms of vascular insufficiency such as angina, claudication or transient ischaemic attacks, or a history of attacks of abdominal pain suggestive of acute pancreatitis.

The past history should include details of any previous measurements of serum lipids and of clinical events such as myocardial infarction or stroke and therapeutic interventions such as coronary artery bypass grafting (CABG), angioplasty and cholecystectomy. A history of diabetes, thyroid dysfunction, gout, gall stones or renal disease is also relevant.

Family history is of great importance, especially the age of onset or death from coronary heart disease (CHD) and the presence of dyslipidaemia in first and second degree relatives. In the US Nurses Health Study the relative risk of manifesting fatal CHD was 5.0 if one or other parent had developed CHD before the age of 60 years. The predictive effect of a family history of CHD is largely independent of other risk factors, implying a separate mechanism,[1] but a family history of other risk factors should also be sought, including hypertension, diabetes and gout. The social history should include details of ethnicity, occupation, marital status and age and sex of any children. Premature CHD is especially common in Asians in whom low levels of high density lipoprotein (HDL) cholesterol and increased Lp(a) are found more frequently than a raised low density lipoprotein (LDL) cholesterol. Lifestyle enquiries should include dietary habits, alcohol, coffee and sucrose intake, current and past smoking habits, amount of exercise taken and details of any current medication.

EXAMINATION

A full physical examination should be undertaken, looking for any obvious facial signs of dyslipidaemia such as corneal arcus and xanthelasma. Additional sites to examine are the palms of the hands, elbows, knees and buttocks for cutaneous xanthomas, and the dorsum of the hands and feet, pretibial tuberosities and Achilles tendons for tendon xanthomas. The significance of these physical signs is discussed below.

Other signs which should be sought are aortic murmurs, carotid and femoral bruits, and the presence of any form of retinopathy. Abdominal examination should include assessment of liver size and, in obese patients, measurement of the waist circumference or waist:hip ratio. Evidence of any endocrinological disorders should also be sought, especially hypothyroidism or Cushing's syndrome. The blood pressure must be measured and the urine tested for protein and glucose. Microalbuminuria should be looked for in diabetics. Also performed routinely are measurements of height and weight, and a resting electrocardiogram on the first visit.

Corneal arcus, xanthelasma and xanthomas

The presence of a corneal arcus before the age of 60 years is often a sign of hypercholesterolaemia (Figure 5.1). It reflects deposition of lipoprotein lipids within the eye and tends to occur more frequently in smokers than in non-smokers. In a study involving over 3000 men, the presence of an arcus was associated with a significantly increased risk of CHD, even after adjusting for serum cholesterol and smoking.[2]

Xanthelasma (Figure 5.2) is a less specific sign of hyperlipidaemia than corneal arcus and is quite often seen in normolipidaemic people. Despite this, however, subtle abnormalities of serum lipids seem relatively common and the frequency of CHD is increased.[3]

Although the existence of corneal arcus and xanthelasma often indicates an associated increase in LDL cholesterol, the fact that these signs can occur in

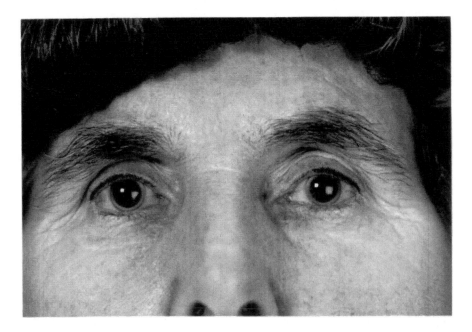

Figure 5.1 Corneal arcus.

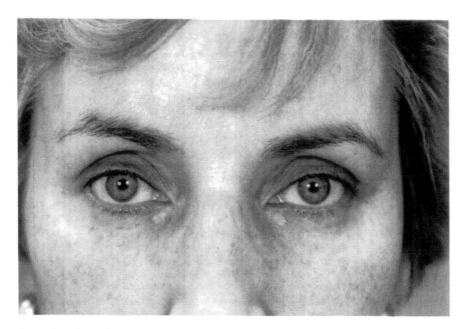

Figure 5.2 Xanthelasma.

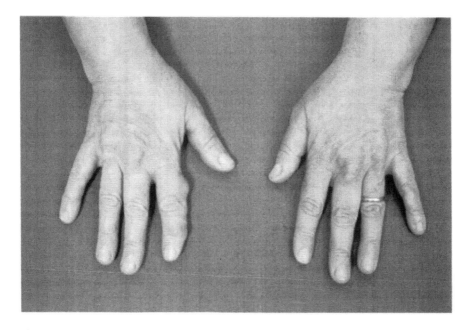

Figure 5.3 Xanthomas in extensor tendons of hands.

normolipidaemic individuals suggests that they may also reflect changes in tissue permeability. An underlying increase in vascular endothelial permeability could explain why corneal arcus and xanthelasma appear to be risk factors in their own right.

Tendon xanthomas are, in the vast majority of patients, a sign of familial hyper-cholesterolaemia (FH) (Figures 5.3 and 5.4). They are age-related, being rare before the age of 20 years but increasingly common thereafter. Two other types of xan-thomas occur which are characteristic of accumulation of cholesterol-rich remnant particles or triglyceride-rich lipoproteins, respectively. Palmar striae, namely yel-lowish discolorations of the normally red creases in the palm of the hand, are virtu-ally pathognomonic of that rare form of mixed hyperlipidaemia known as 'type III' (Figure 5.5). In contrast, eruptive xanthomas typically occur in severe hypertriglyc-eridaemia, especially on the back and buttocks (Figure 5.6). Both these forms of cutaneous xanthoma disappear rapidly after appropriate lipid-lowering therapy, whereas tendon xanthomas take much longer to resolve.

LABORATORY TESTS

Assuming that initial screening revealed a raised non-fasted serum total cholesterol, a second sample of serum or plasma should be obtained after an overnight fast of at least ten hours. Measurements should include total cholesterol, triglyceride and HDL cholesterol, with calculation of LDL cholesterol and the total:HDL cholesterol ratio as described below. If possible, Lp(a) should also be measured. In addition to characterizing the severity and nature of the patient's dyslipidaemia, a search

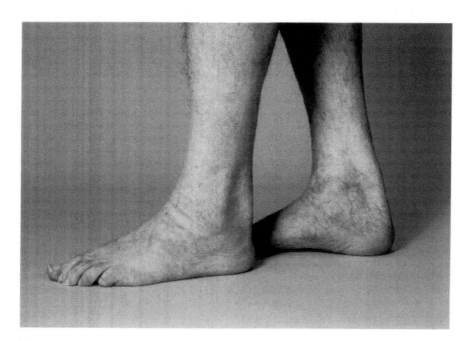

Figure 5.4 Xanthomas in Achilles tendons.

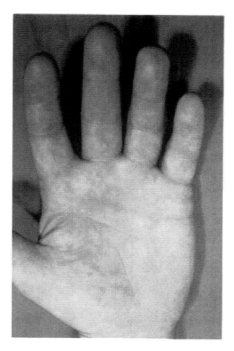

Figure 5.5 Palmar striae, best seen in the upper horizontal crease.

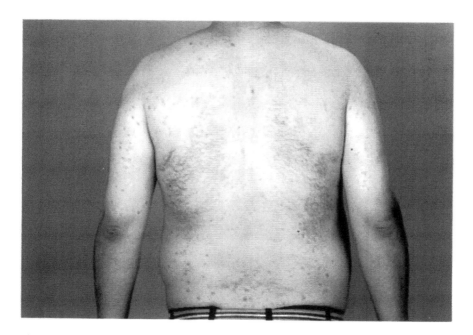

Figure 5.6 Eruptive xanthomas on back and over triceps.

should be made for underlying causes. This involves routinely undertaking bio-chemical tests of renal and hepatic function, including γ-glutamyl transpeptidase (which, if raised, is often an index of excess alcohol intake), fasting glucose and thyroid function tests (tetraiodothyronine and thyroid-stimulating hormone). Additional investigations, which may require referral to a specialist centre, include apoE phenotyping and assessment of LDL particle size and density.

Calculation of LDL cholesterol and total:HDL cholesterol ratio

Lipoprotein concentrations in plasma or serum are usually expressed in terms of their cholesterol content, determined after preliminary isolation of very low density lipoprotein (VLDL) by ultracentrifugation. In routine clinical practice, however, ultracentrifugation is seldom performed and instead values for VLDL and LDL cholesterol are derived by applying the formula of Friedewald et al.[4] This is based on assumptions that most of the triglyceride in fasting plasma is located in VLDL and that the molar ratio of triglyceride to cholesterol in VLDL is 2.19:1, except in patients with type III hyperlipoproteinaemia or marked hypertriglyceridaemia (>4.5 mmol/L), for whom the formula is inaccurate. Apart from these exceptions, it provides a reasonably accurate means of calculating LDL cholesterol:

$$LDLC = TC - HDLC - \frac{TG}{2.2} \text{ (mmol/L)}$$

where LDLC = LDL cholesterol, TC = total cholesterol, HDLC = HDL cholesterol and TG = triglyceride. (The divisor for triglyceride is 5 if the values are expressed in mg/dl).

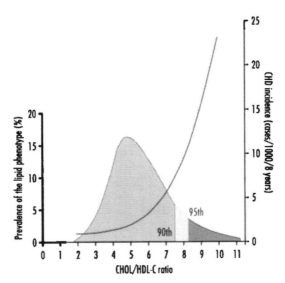

Figure 5.7 Frequency distribution of total:HDL cholesterol ratios and their relationship (red trace) with the incidence of coronary heart disease (CHD) in PROCAM. Chol, total cholesterol; HDL-C, high density lipoprotein cholesterol. Reproduced with permission from International Task Force for Prevention of CHD/IAS. In *Nutrition, Metabolism and Cardiovascular Disease* 1998; 8:205–71.

The use of calculated LDL cholesterol values when assessing CHD risk underlines the importance of high degrees of accuracy and precision in laboratory measurement of total and HDL cholesterol and triglyceride. LDL cholesterol will be underestimated if a non-fasting triglyceride value is used in the Friedewald formula.

The opposing influences of total and HDL cholesterol have led to the use of the ratio of one to the other as a predictor of risk and the total:HDL cholesterol ratio was second only to the Framingham logistic model in its ability to predict CHD risk in over 3000 men and women followed up for 12 years.[5] In the PROCAM study the incidence of CHD increased steeply in men with a ratio greater than 5 (Figure 5.7).

ELECTROCARDIOGRAPHIC ABNORMALITIES

Evidence of a previous myocardial infarction (often silent) on a resting electrocardiogram (ECG) is strongly associated with risk of recurrent infarction or CHD death.[6] Left ventricular hypertrophy (LVH) on the ECG also increases CHD risk, and although its prevalence is less than 2% in young adults, this rises to approximately 10% in elderly individuals. The presence of LVH increases CHD risk 7.5 times in men and 5 times in women below the age of 65 years.[7]

Several other ECG abnormalities are associated with increased CHD risk including bundle branch block,[8] non-specific S–T segment and T wave changes[9] and premature ventricular contractions.[10] In the 29 years follow-up of the Chicago Western Electric Study, minor ST–T abnormalities were associated with a relative risk of fatal CHD of 1.4 and major ECG changes with a relative risk of >2.[11]

QUANTIFICATION OF CORONARY HEART DISEASE RISK

As discussed in Chapter 2 therapeutic management decisions in dyslipidaemic patients are increasingly based on an assessment of absolute risk of CHD, which reflects all the major risk factors, rather than on serum lipids alone. However, as previously stated, total and HDL cholesterol are probably the most important risk factors for CHD in epidemiological studies.[12] The total cholesterol level is a useful indicator in younger people, but it loses some of its strength after the age of 55 years, especially in men. In contrast, HDL cholesterol retains its predictive power up to the age of 80 years.

Cigarette smoking has greater strength as a risk factor in men than in women, probably because male smokers usually smoke more, but women who smoke 20 cigarettes per day have a greatly increased risk for CHD as compared with non-smoking women.

In determining CHD risk attributable to blood pressure, systolic pressure measurement is used, because it has been found to be more highly predictive of future vascular disease than diastolic pressure.[13]

Glucose intolerance is a stronger CHD risk factor for women than for men according to Framingham data. Women seldom develop CHD before the menopause, unless they have glucose intolerance or an inherited form of dyslipidaemia such as FH.

Multiple logistic model to calculate risk

Sixteen-year follow-up data from the Framingham study were converted to a 6-year CHD rate, which was then related to risk factors at entry.[12] Using a multiple logistic model, parameters were estimated for age, plasma cholesterol, systolic blood pressure, cigarette smoking, LVH on the electrocardiogram and glucose intolerance, based on regressed data of CHD incidence for both sexes. A quadratic term, age × age, and the cross-product, cholesterol × age, improved the fit of incidence data and the original 6-year CHD equations were modified with an HDL cholesterol logistic parameter derived from subsequent follow-up data. This enabled the risk of CHD to be calculated for men aged 35–65 years and women aged 45–65 years, based on presence or absence of cigarette smoking, LVH and glucose intolerance, as well as on levels of total cholesterol (over the range 4.65–8.7 mmol/L), HDL cholesterol (range 0.8–1.7 mmol/L and 1.0–1.8 mmol/L for men and women, respectively) and systolic blood pressure (range 105–195 mmHg). Comparison with the PROCAM risk algorithm showed that the latter was marginally better as a risk predictor than the Framingham score but both tended to overestimate risk in British men.[14]

The coefficients used in the risk factor equations for men and women can be used to program calculators or small desk-top computers and provide a convenient means of quantifying the overall risk of CHD. Predictability of CHD might be improved to some extent by inclusion of risk factors such as family history and Lp(a),[14] but even when all the known risk factors are taken into account this explains only 50% of the variability in risk between individuals.

Limitations of risk assessment

As indicated above, estimating the risk of developing clinical manifestations of CHD within a given period of time is, at best, informed guesswork, because individuals vary so much in their susceptibility to factors which cause CHD. All data on risk factors are derived from groups of people and therefore reflect averages, often with wide confidence limits. Despite these caveats, estimation of risk is an integral part of CHD prevention, especially because there is now evidence that effective intervention can not only decrease future risk, but also arrest, or even reverse, established disease.

At this stage it is worth stressing again the distinction between absolute and relative risk. Absolute risk defines the expected rate of CHD events for any given combination of age, sex and other risk factors, whereas relative risk is the ratio between the absolute risk in an individual and someone of the same age and sex who has no other risk factors. For example, young people with heterozygous FH have a high relative risk but a low absolute risk. On the other hand, with increasing age absolute risk rises but relative risk falls, a reflection of how common CHD is after the age of 65 years.

Whichever method or criterion is used, however, it is impossible to be certain whether or not a given individual will develop CHD. For example, two-thirds of asymptomatic men aged 40–55 years in the highest quintiles of blood pressure and cholesterol remain free of CHD for the next 25 years.[15] Thus, the majority of those who are theoretically at high risk may be treated unnecessarily. The likelihood of this is, of course, reduced to nil if evidence of clinically unapparent CHD can be obtained. Therefore, it makes sense to search for pre-clinical vascular disease in those at risk, using one or more of the non-invasive methods described below.

NON-INVASIVE INDICES OF PRE-CLINICAL VASCULAR DISEASE

Methods currently available for detecting pre-clinical or silent atherosclerosis can be divided into those that identify abnormalities of vascular structure and those that provide evidence of vascular or myocardial dysfunction. Non-invasive methods of assessing the presence and severity of atherosclerosis are ultrasound examination of the carotid and femoral arteries, and computed tomographic (CT) scanning for coronary calcification. Non-invasive methods used to detect myocardial ischaemia or vascular dysfunction include exercise electrocardiography, measurement of the ankle:arm blood pressure ratio and flow-mediated arterial dilatation. Evidence that the presence of pre-clinical disease predicts an increased risk of CHD has come from the Cardiovascular Health Study in which asymptomatic individuals over the age of 65 years with an abnormal carotid ultrasound examination, reduced ankle:arm pressure ratio or major electrocardiographic abnormality were shown to have a relative risk of developing coronary events that was double that of individuals without these abnormalities.[16] Similar findings were reported recently from the Rotterdam Study.[17]

Carotid ultrasound

A correlation between atherosclerosis in coronary and carotid arteries has long been recognized in post-mortem studies. Furthermore, coronary angiography in over 500 patients with clinical evidence of carotid artery disease revealed severe coronary lesions in 35% of them.[18] More recently, a number of studies have explored this relationship using high resolution B-mode carotid ultrasound. The extent of carotid disease is greater in patients with known coronary artery disease than in controls.[19] Conversely, a large prospective study has shown that the severity of carotid abnormalities on ultrasound is a powerful predictor of the risk of acute myocardial infarction,[20] the presence of a stenotic plaque being associated with a sixfold higher risk than in those with no abnormalities. The presence and severity of carotid abnormalities were positively correlated with LDL cholesterol and negatively correlated with HDL cholesterol.[21] Other studies showed a good correlation between carotid intimal-medial thickness and the cholesterol × years score[22] (Figure 5.8).

Carotid intimal-medial thickness increased by 0.13 mm over 2 years in untreated patients, and was correlated with age, smoking and LDL cholesterol.[23] Reversal of

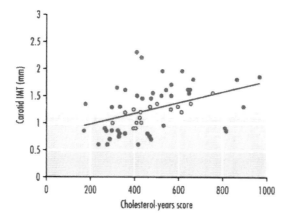

Figure 5.8 Correlation between carotid intimal-medial thickness (IMT) and cholesterol years score in 59 familial hypercholesterolaemia heterozygotes. Reproduced with permission from Sidhu et al.[22]

this process has been demonstrated in a number of lipid-lowering trials.[24,25] Thus carotid ultrasound findings provide a surrogate for both the probable presence and the response to therapy of coronary artery disease.

Computed tomographic measurement of coronary calcification

The use of electron beam computed tomographic (EBCT) scanning for detecting coronary calcification was reviewed recently.[26] The coronary calcification score (CCS) has been shown to correlate strongly with the presence and severity of coronary atherosclerosis, both on histological and angiographic criteria, and has been proposed as a means of determining the need for risk factor modification. However, concerns have been expressed about the relatively low specificity of coronary calcification, lack of evidence that it provides additional information to Framingham-based estimates of risk, and the paucity of prospective data relating the CCS to CHD events. Another limitation has been the cost of the EBCT scanners. Recently, however, multi-slice CT scanners have been shown to produce comparable calcium scores, promising greater availability, and several publications have demonstrated the predictive power of the CCS for CHD events.

Kondos et al[27] followed 5635 asymptomatic individuals for 37 months after an EBCT scan and found significant differences in myocardial infarction and in the need for revascularization procedures between men with an age and sex related score >75th percentile and those with a score in the 1–74th percentile range. Overall the presence of coronary calcification was associated with relative risks of a CHD event of 10.5 in men and 2.6 in women, significantly greater than those associated with any of the conventional risk factors, apart from age in men.

In a second study 102 patients under the age of 60, mostly men, had an EBCT scan within two weeks of a first myocardial infarction and before any form of intervention.[28] Of these, 61% had a CCS greater than the 90th percentile, compared with

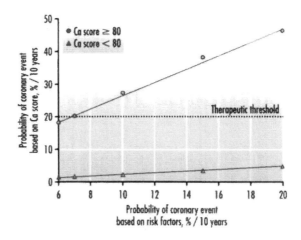

Figure 5.9 Influence of coronary calcification (Ca) score on probability of coronary events based on risk factors estimates. Reproduced from The Lancet, 363, Thompson GR, Partridge J, Coronary calcification score: the coronary-risk impact factor, 557–9, 2004, with permission from Elsevier.[26]

only 6% of matched controls ($P = 0.001$). This differential was most marked in those less than 35 years old and in 90% of instances the culprit vessel was calcified.

Several studies have shown correlations between coronary calcification and conventional risk factors but most of the variation in calcification scores among individuals remains unexplained by differences in their risk factors. Further evidence of the anomalous relationship between CHD risk factors and coronary calcification has come from a study that analysed published data to compare Framingham-derived estimates of CHD risk with estimates based on the CCS.[29] The authors calculated that for any given pre-test probability of a CHD event, based on risk factors, having a calcification score of ≥80 would triple the probability whereas having a score of <80 would reduce it by a factor of 5. As shown in Figure 5.9, if the threshold for risk factor modification is set at 20% / 10 years, then virtually all individuals at intermediate risk (6–20% / 10 years) qualify for treatment if their calcification score is ≥80, whereas none do if their score is <80.

Discrepancies between the calcification score and Framingham-based estimates of risk presumably reflect the differing susceptibility of individuals to their prevailing risk factors, implying that the coronary calcification score reflects the overall impact of risk factors, known and unknown, on the arterial wall. Combining the two approaches should enable clinicians to assess better the management of asymptomatic patients, as was recognized in the latest European guidelines on cardiovascular disease prevention[30] (see Chapter 6).

Exercise testing

Stress testing, using exercise electrocardiography, is a theoretically attractive means of detecting subclinical myocardial ischaemia, yet its yield is very low when used in asymptomatic people and false-positive tests are common. In the Lipid Research Clinics Program the frequency of positive exercise tests was similar in hyperlipidaemic and normolipidaemic individuals at 6.2% and 5.4%, respectively.[31] Thus exercise testing is probably best reserved for patients with chest pain of uncertain origin and asymptomatic patients with FH,[32] in whom the yield of positive tests is higher.

Flow-mediated arterial dilatation

The importance of endothelium-dependent modulation of vascular tone is now well recognized. Evidence that endothelial cells release mediators which induce vasodilatation stemmed from the discovery of prostacyclin. Following this, it was shown that the vasodilatory effect of acetylcholine was dependent on the release from intact endothelium of a compound containing nitric oxide, biosynthesized from L-arginine.

A non-invasive method of assessing vascular endothelial function was originally developed for use in children and later applied to adults.[33] This involves measurement of the diameter of the brachial artery (or femoral artery in children) by ultrasound before and after a period of ischaemia, induced by inflating a sphygmomanometer cuff, release of which causes reactive hyperaemia with a transient enhancement of blood flow and increased endothelial shear stress. In those with normal endothelial function this results in an approximate 10% increase in brachial artery diameter. Absent or reduced dilatation was observed in hypercholesterolaemic children and adults, and in patients who smoked or had coronary artery disease. This convenient test not only provides a sensitive and reproducible means of assessing vascular endothelial function in individuals with an increased risk of CHD, but can also be used to monitor therapeutic response to interventions directed at the underlying risk factors.

REFERENCES

1. Thompson GR. Screening relatives of patients with premature coronary heart disease. Heart 2002; 87:390–4.
2. Rosenman RH, Brand RJ, Scholtz RI et al. Relation of corneal arcus to cardiovascular risk factors and the incidence of coronary disease. N Engl J Med 1974; 291:1322–4.
3. Watanabe A, Yoshmura A, Wakasugi T et al. Serum lipids, lipoprotein lipids and coronary heart disease in patients with xanthelasma palpebrarum. Atherosclerosis 1981; 38:283–90.
4. Friedewald WT, Levy RI, Fredrickson DS. Estimation of the concentration of low-density lipoprotein cholesterol in plasma, without use of the preparative ultracentrifuge. Clin Chem 1972; 18:499–502.
5. Grover SA, Coupal L, Hu X-P. Identifying adults at increased risk of coronary disease. J Am Med Assoc 1995; 274:801–6.
6. Kannel WB, Abbott RD. Incidence and prognosis of unrecognized myocardial infarction: an update of the Framingham Study. N Engl J Med 1984; 311:1144–7.
7. Kannell WB, Dannenberg AL, Levy D. Population implications of electrocardiographic left ventricular hypertrophy. Am J Cardiol 1987; 60 (Suppl):851–931.
8. Kannel WB. Common electrocardiographic markers for subsequent clinical coronary events. Circulation 1987; 75(Suppl 2):25–7.
9. Kreger BE, Kannel WB, Cupples LA. Electrocardiographic precursors of sudden unexpected death: the Framingham Study. Circulation 1987; 75(Suppl 2):22–4.
10. Knutsen R, Knutsen SF, Curb JD et al. The predictive value of resting electrocardiograms for 12-year incidence of coronary heart disease in the Honolulu Heart Program. J Clin Epidemiol 1988; 41:293–302.
11. Daviglus ML, Liao Y, Greenland P et al. Association of nonspecific minor ST-T abnormalities with cardiovascular mortality: the Chicago Western Electric Study. J Am Med Assoc 1999; 281:530–6.
12. Wilson PWF, Castelli WP, Kannel WB. Coronary risk prediction in adults (The Framingham Heart Study). Am J Cardiol 1987; 59:91G–4G.
13. Stamler J, Neaton JD, Wentworth DN. Blood pressure (systolic and diastolic) and risk of fatal coronary heart disease. Hypertension 1989; 13(Suppl I):I2–I12.
14. Cooper JA, Miller GJ, Humphries SE. A comparison of the PROCAM and Framingham point-scoring systems for estimation of individual risk of coronary heart disease in the Second Northwick Park Heart Study. Atherosclerosis 2005; 181:93–100.
15. Naylor CD, Basinski A, Frank JW et al. Asymptomatic hypercholesterolemia: a clinical policy review. J Clin Epidemiol 1990; 43:1029–121.
16. Kuller LH, Shemanski L, Psaty BM et al. Subclinical disease as an independent risk factor for cardiovascular disease. Circulation 1995; 92:720–6.
17. Van der Meer IM, Bots ML, Hofman A et al. Predictive value of non-invasive measures of atherosclerosis for incident myocardial infarction: the Rotterdam Study. Circulation 2004; 109: 1089–94.
18. Hertzer NR, Young JR, Beven EG et al. Coronary angiography in 506 patients with extracranial cerebrovascular disease. Arch Intern Med 1985; 145:849–52.
19. Howard G, Ryu JE, Evans GW et al. Extracranial carotid atherosclerosis in patients with and without transient ischemic attacks and coronary artery disease. Arteriosclerosis 1990; 10:714–19.

20. Salonen JT, Salonen R. Ultrasonographically assessed carotid morphology and the risk of coronary heart disease. Arterioscler Thromb 1991; 11:1245–9.
21. Salonen R, Seppännen K, Rauramaa R et al. Prevalence of carotid atherosclerosis and serum cholesterol levels in Eastern Finland. Arteriosclerosis 1988; 8:788–92.
22. Sidhu PS, Naoumova RP, Maher VMG et al. The extracranial carotid artery in familial hypercholesterolaemia: relationship of intimal-medial thickness and plaque morphology with plasma lipids and coronary heart disease. J Cardiovasc Risk 1996; 3:61–7.
23. Salonen R, Salonen JT. Progression of carotid atherosclerosis and its determinants: a population-based ultrasonography study. Atherosclerosis 1990; 81:33–40.
24. Furberg CD, Adams HP Jr, Applegate WB et al for the Asymptomatic Carotid Artery Progression Study (ACAPS) Research Group. Effect of lovastatin on early carotid atherosclerosis and cardiovascular events. Circulation 1994; 90:1679–87.
25. Crouse JR III, Byington RP, Bond MG et al. Pravastatin, lipids, and atherosclerosis in the carotid arteries (PLAC II). Am J Cardiol 1995; 75:455–9.
26. Thompson GR, Partridge J. Coronary calcification score: the coronary-risk impact factor. Lancet 2004; 363:557–9.
27. Kondos GT, Hoff JA, Sevrukov A et al. Electron-beam tomography coronary artery calcium and cardiac events: a 37-month follow-up of 5635 initially asymptomatic low- to intermediate-risk adults. Circulation 2003; 107:2571–6.
28. Pohle K, Ropers D, Maffert R et al. Coronary calcifications in young patients with first, unheralded myocardial infarction: a risk factor matched analysis by electron beam tomography. Heart 2003; 89:625–8.
29. Greenland P, Gaziano JM. Selecting asymptomatic patients for coronary computed tomography or electrocardiographic exercise testing. N Engl J Med 2003; 349:465–73.
30. De Backer G, Abrosioni E, Borch-Johnsen K et al. Executive summary: European guidelines on cardiovascular disease prevention in clinical practice. Third Joint Task Force of European and other societies on cardiovascular disease prevention in clinical practice. Eur Heart J 2003; 24:1601–10.
31. Gordon DJ, Ekelund L-G, Karon JM et al. Predictive value of the exercise tolerance test for mortality in North American men: the Lipid Research Clinics Mortality Follow-up Study. Circulation 1986; 74:252–61.
32. Civeira F and International Panel on Management of Familial Hypercholesterolemia. Guidelines for the diagnosis and management of heterozygous familial hypercholesterolemia. Atherosclerosis 2004; 173:55–68.
33. Celermajer DS, Sorensen KE, Gooch VM et al. Non-invasive detection of endothelial dysfunction in children and adults at risk of atherosclerosis. Lancet 1992; 340:1111–15.

6

Guidelines for the management of dyslipidaemia

INTRODUCTION

The current emphasis on evidence-based medicine has made guidelines a necessary evil of our time. This description is used advisedly, not only because of the confusing multiplicity of guidelines published at international, national, regional and local level, but also because they exemplify for many the increasing regimentation of medical practice. Knowledge of guidelines is now part of the Consultant Appraisal process in the UK, and failure to adhere to them could leave a physician open to criticism. Seen from another angle, however, guidelines provide practical advice to the generalist in an age of ever-increasing specialization and help maintain the standard of health care.

Over the last 30 years or so, guidance on the prevention of coronary heart disease (CHD) by dietary means has been issued by governmental and professional organizations in many Western countries, including the reports on Diet and Coronary Heart Disease by the Committee on Medical Aspects of Food Policy (COMA), published by the Department of Health and Social Security in Britain in 1974, 1984 and 1994. The most recent of these recommended that the average contribution of total fat to dietary energy should not exceed 35%, of which not more than 10% should be saturated fat, 10% polyunsaturated fat and less than 2% trans fatty acids.[1] Other recommendations included maintaining intake of dietary cholesterol below 250 mg/day and increasing the consumption of ω-3 fatty acids to 200 mg/day.

The first guidelines for the medical profession on the prevention of CHD in the UK were published in 1976 in the form of a Joint Report from the Royal College of Physicians and the British Cardiac Society,[2] which dealt with the management of the major risk factors known at the time. However, despite acknowledgement of the need to treat hypercholesterolaemia, the focus of the report was on dietary measures and the use of lipid-lowering drugs was given only a perfunctory mention. In the light of subsequent events, discussed below, this turns out to have been a fortuitous lapse.

The clofibrate saga

In 1978, the results of the World Health Organization (WHO) primary prevention trial of clofibrate were published, which showed that although clofibrate decreased the incidence of non-fatal myocardial infarcts this was offset by an increase in gastrointestinal disorders, especially gallstones.[3] A subsequent analysis of over 9 years of in-trial and post-trial follow-up data revealed that clofibrate-treated patients had sustained a 25% increase in total mortality;[4] this caused the Committee on the Safety of Medicines to issue a warning, which resulted in the virtual cessation of clofibrate prescribing in the UK and cast a shadow over lipid-lowering policies in general.

The uncertainties resulting from the WHO trial persisted until 1984, when the successful outcome of the Lipid Research Clinics Primary Prevention Trial of cholestyramine[5] led to a renewal of confidence in the relevance and safety of cholesterol-lowering measures to the prevention of CHD.

GUIDELINES ISSUED IN THE PRE-STATIN ERA

The year 1985 saw the award of the Nobel Prize to Goldstein and Brown for their discovery of the receptor for low density lipoprotein (LDL), and also publication of the recommendations of the Consensus Conference on Lowering Blood Cholesterol to Prevent Heart Disease.[6] The latter summarized the evidence linking cholesterol and CHD, defined risk of CHD according to the severity of hypercholesterolaemia, and provided advice on dietary and drug treatment. This authoritative statement, issued under the aegis of the National Institutes of Health in Bethesda, set the standard for all guidelines published over the next few years, which included two from the British Hyperlipidaemia Association[7,8] and three from the European Atherosclerosis Society.[9-11]

In 1988, the National Cholesterol Education Program (NCEP) Expert Panel published the first of its reports on the management of hypercholesterolaemia in the USA.[12] This provided detailed recommendations on the levels of plasma cholesterol, specifically LDL cholesterol, at which treatment should be initiated, as well as the target levels to be achieved by diet and, if necessary, drugs.

The recommendations in 1994 of the Task Force set up by the European Societies of Cardiology and Hypertension and the European Atherosclerosis Society[13] were novel in that they included estimation of absolute risk of CHD as an index of when to treat dyslipidaemia in the context of primary prevention. Estimates of absolute risk were based on the Framingham model but omitted high density lipoprotein (HDL) cholesterol as a variable.

CURRENT GUIDELINES

All the guidelines in current use were drafted after the publication of the Scandinavian Simvastatin Survival Study (4S) in 1994, which provided clear proof that lowering LDL cholesterol reduced both total and coronary mortality.[14] However, guidelines drafted before that date had to take account of the controversy then prevalent as to whether lowering serum cholesterol led to an increase in noncardiovascular mortality.

Suspicions that lipid-lowering therapy induced an increase in noncardiovascular causes of death such as cancer had been observed in individuals on diets high in polyunsaturated fat[15] and, as mentioned previously, the WHO investigators reported that clofibrate increased morbidity and mortality from a range of disorders, particularly those reflecting the drug's action in promoting biliary cholesterol secretion. This led Oliver to question the validity of lowering serum cholesterol as a means of preventing CHD and to imply that cholesterol lowering per se, whether by diet or drugs, might be unsafe.[16] Support for this argument was provided by a meta-analysis of prevention trials, which concluded that cholesterol-lowering increased the incidence of accidental deaths, including murder and suicide.[17] One of the trials reported a significant excess of deaths from fractures, drug reactions, burns, foreign bodies, tooth extractions, freezing, heat-stroke, drowning and suicide but, as was later pointed out, it was difficult to conceive of a causal mechanism whereby cholesterol reduction could have so many disparate effects.[18]

The issue was resolved by both the reassuring results of the 4S study and a meta-analysis of 40 published studies relating non-cardiovascular causes of death to serum cholesterol.[19] Apart from an unexplained increase in haemorrhagic stroke in individuals with high blood pressure and low cholesterol, no evidence was found that lowering cholesterol increased mortality from any cause. The observed associations between cancer and suicide and low serum cholesterol were attributed to confounding, in that a low serum cholesterol is often a consequence of cancer and can also occur in depressed individuals who neglect themselves.

US guidelines

The Third Report of the NCEP (Adult Treatment Panel III) resembled its predecessors[12,20] but placed increased emphasis on the primary prevention of CHD and re-defined the level at which a low HDL cholesterol constitutes a risk factor.[21] It retained the use of the LDL cholesterol level as the criterion of both treatment initiation and therapeutic goal: the greater the risk of CHD, the lower the level of LDL cholesterol at which treatment is initiated and the lower the target level to be achieved. Patients with CHD, diabetes or multiple risk factors, including hypertriglyceridaemia, are regarded as being at greatest risk of a CHD event, and the majority of them will require lipid-lowering drug therapy to achieve the target LDL cholesterol of 2.6 mmol/L. However, lifestyle changes, including diet and exercise, may achieve the less stringent LDL cholesterol targets recommended for those at lesser risk.

In addition to risk factors other than the level of LDL cholesterol (Table 6.1), several inherited forms of dyslipidaemia predispose to premature CHD, namely familial hypercholesterolaemia, familial combined hyperlipidaemia and severe polygenic hypercholesterolaemia (LDL cholesterol >5.7 mmol/L). So too does the metabolic syndrome, characterized by abdominal obesity, insulin resistance and dyslipidaemia, as defined in Table 6.2. In contrast, a raised HDL cholesterol (≥1.6 mmol/L) is regarded as a negative risk factor and should be subtracted when determining the risk category. Risk is quantified with a Framingham-based point scoring system and those estimated to have a >20% / 10 years risk, and diabetics, are regarded as being at equivalent risk to individuals with CHD, and therefore in need of equally stringent therapeutic intervention.

Since the publication of ATP III in 2001 the results of several major statin trials have been published, including the Heart Protection Study.[22] This large trial investigated the effects on mortality and morbidity of cholesterol-lowering therapy in patients with or at high risk of cardiovascular disease. Men and women aged 40–80 years with a total cholesterol of >3.5 mmol/L were randomized to receive either simvastatin at 40 mg daily, antioxidant vitamins, the two combined or placebo. Patients allocated to simvastatin had decreases in total and cardiovascular mortality of 12% and 17%, respectively, and decreases in CHD events and strokes of 26% and

---

Table 6.1   Major risk factors for coronary heart disease (CHD), except LDL cholesterol and diabetes[21]

- Age (men ≥45 years; women ≥55 years)
- Cigarette smoking
- Hypertension (≥140/90 mmHg or on antihypertensive medication)
- Family history of premature CHD (in male first-degree relative <55 years or in female first-degree relative <65 years)
- Low HDL cholesterol (<1 mmol/L or 40 mg/dl)
- High HDL cholesterol (>1.55 mmol/L or 60 mg/dl) acts as a 'negative' risk factor
- Metabolic syndrome

Table 6.2   Diagnostic criteria of the metabolic syndrome[21]

Any three of:	Men	Women
Waist (cm)	>102	>88
HDL-C (mmol/L)	<1	<1.3
TG (mmol/L)	≥1.7	
BP (mmHg)	≥130/85	
Fasting glucose (mmol/L)	≥6.1	

HDL-C, high density lipoprotein cholesterol; TG, triglyceride; BP, blood pressure.

27%. Benefit from simvastatin occurred irrespective of the level of LDL cholesterol at entry; one-third of the patients had a baseline value below 3 mmol/L, which suggests that high-risk individuals should be treated with simvastatin at 40 mg/day, or its equivalent, irrespective of their LDL cholesterol level. These results and those of subsequent trials have endorsed the concept 'the lower the LDL, the better' (see Chapter 8) and have led the NCEP to propose modifications to the original ATP III guidelines,[23] as shown in Table 6.3. Physicians are given the option of starting drug therapy at LDL levels below those in the original guidelines and of achieving lower LDL or non-HDL cholesterol goals, as appropriate, in high-risk patients.

The practical application of ATP III in a clinical context is discussed in Chapter 7.

International guidelines

The self-appointed International Task Force for Prevention of Coronary Heart Disease co-operated with the International Atherosclerosis Society to produce a set of guidelines which were published in 1998.[24] Like the first Joint European Societies guidelines,[13] estimation of overall ('global') risk of CHD is used to determine the need for preventive therapy. However, instead of the Framingham model, the International Guidelines use the PROCAM algorithm, derived from the Munster Heart Study. This takes account not only of age, smoking, systolic blood pressure, diabetes and HDL cholesterol, but also the presence of angina, a family history of myocardial infarction, and LDL cholesterol and triglyceride. Estimates of risk obtained using the Framingham and PROCAM algorithms have been shown to correlate well in British patients,[25] but although these guidelines contain some useful information they are too complicated to use in clinical practice.

Table 6.3 ATP III LDL-cholesterol cut-points and goals, with proposed modifications based on recent clinical trials shown in red[23]

Risk category	Initiate therapeutic lifestyle changes if LDL-C:	Consider drug therapy if LDL-C:	LDL-C goal
High risk CHD or CHD risk equivalents (10-year risk >20%)	2.6 mmol/L	2.6 mmol/L Optional if <2.6 mmol/L (<100 mg/dl)	2.6 mmol/L Option: <1.8 mmol/L (<70 mg/dl)
Moderately high risk ≥2 risk factors (10-year risk 10–20%)	3.4 mmol/L	≥ 3.4 mmol/L Optional if 2.6–3.3 mmol/L (100–130 mg/dl)	<3.4 mmol/L
Moderate risk ≥2 risk factors (10-year risk <10%)	≥ 3.4 mmol/L	≥ 4.1 mmol/L	<3.4 mmol/L
Lower risk 0–1 risk factor	≥ 4.1 mmol/L	≥ 4.9 mmol/L Optional if 4.1–4.8 mmol/L (160–185 mg/dl)	<4.1 mmol/L

[a] or non-HDL-C <2.6 mmol/L (100 mg/dl) if hypertriglyceridaemic. LDL-C, low density lipoprotein cholesterol; for other abbreviations, see tables and text.

Joint European societies' guidelines

The third set of joint guidelines published by the European Societies of Cardiology and Hypertension, and the European Atherosclerosis Society[26] differs radically from its predecessors[13,27] in proposing a new way of estimating risk: the Systematic Coronary Risk Evaluation (SCORE) system, which grades risk in terms of the 10-year risk of fatal cardiovascular disease (CVD) end-points. As shown in Figure 6.1, CVD risk ranges from <1% to ≥15%, separate charts being used for countries in Europe regarded as at low risk (Belgium, France, Greece, Italy, Luxembourg, Spain and Portugal) or at high risk of CVD (all other European countries, including the UK). Risk in individuals is determined by correlating on the relevant chart their age, gender, smoking status, systolic blood pressure and total:HDL cholesterol ratio or total cholesterol. Qualifying factors which increase risk above values shown on the charts include: pre-clinical evidence of atherosclerosis (see Chapter 5); a strong family history of premature CVD and presence of low HDL cholesterol (<1 mmol/L in men or <1.2 mmol/L in women); impaired glucose tolerance; or raised levels of C-reactive protein, fibrinogen, homocysteine, and apoproteins apoB or Lp(a).

High risk is defined as having: established CVD or a CVD risk of ≥5% / 10 years, at current age or if extrapolated to 60 years; markedly raised levels of total (≥8 mmol/L) or LDL cholesterol (≥6 mmol/L); blood pressure ≥180/110 mmHg; or diabetes.

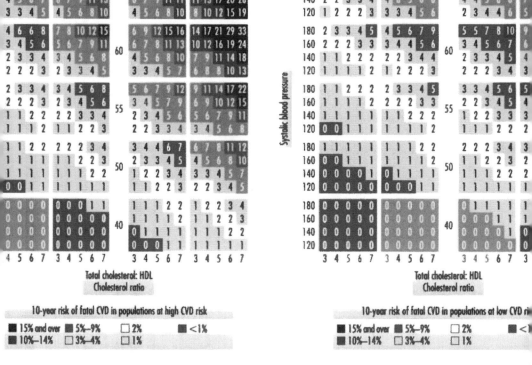

E charts for calculating risk of fatal CVD/10 years for high (left) and low (right) risk regions of Europe according stolic blood pressure and total:HDL cholesterol ratio (reproduced from Ref. 26 with permission).

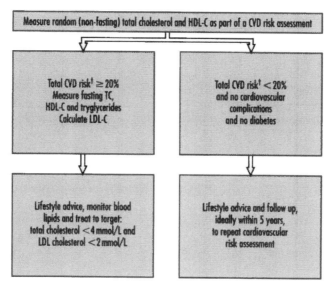

Figure 6.2 Risk thresholds and target levels for cholesterol applicable to asymptomatic patients without CVD in JBS2. [†]Assessed with CVD risk chart. Reproduced with permission.[28]

Management of serum lipids in asymptomatic patients depends upon their estimated risk of CVD. Lifestyle advice includes limiting fat intake to 30% of energy, of which not more than one-third is saturated, and cholesterol intake to <300 mg/day. Total and LDL cholesterol goals are <5 and <3 mmol/L respectively. High-risk individuals may require drug therapy if these goals are not achieved after 3 months of lifestyle change. In those remaining at high risk despite drug therapy, total and LDL cholesterol goals should be lowered to <4.5 and <2.5 mmol/L, respectively.

Joint British Societies' guidelines

The second set of guidelines to be issued by the Joint British Societies on the prevention of cardiovascular disease (JBS2) have recently been published.[28] These differ from their predecessors in emphasizing that preventive measures should be focused equally on individuals with established CVD, diabetics and asymptomatic patients at high risk (CVD risk ≥20% / 10 years, equivalent to a CHD risk of 15% / 10 years), thus doing away with the distinction between primary and secondary prevention. Unacceptably high levels of single risk factors, notably a systolic blood pressure ≥160 mm or diastolic ≥100 mm and a total HDL cholesterol ratio ≥6 come into the same category, as does genetic dyslipidaemia (FH and FCH).

Estimation of total cardiovascular risk (CHD plus stroke but excluding transient ischaemic attack) is based on predictive charts, which take into account age, gender, smoking, systolic blood pressure and total:HDL cholesterol ratio; this should be undertaken opportunistically in all adults ≥40 years, or younger if they have a family history of premature CVD. Screening of first degree relatives of patients with FH or FCH has an even higher priority. Other risk factors not included in the charts are ethnicity (being Asian increases risk ×1.5), abdominal obesity, impaired glucose tolerance, fasting triglyceride >1.7 mmol/L and family history of CVD in a first degree relative, which increases risk × 1.3. In younger persons risk estimates should be extrapolated to age 49 years rather than 60 years, which may be too late to start preventive measures.

The screening protocol, thresholds for intervention and target levels of lipids advocated by JBS2 are shown in Figure 6.2. Optimal levels to be achieved are total cholesterol <4 mmol/L and LDL cholesterol <2 mmol/L, or decreases of 25% and 30%, respectively. Audit (minimum) levels are total cholesterol <5 mmol/L and LDL cholesterol <3 mmol/L, values which were considered as optimal in the previous guidelines.

Multifactorial risk factor management involves lifestyle changes, including increased consumption of plant sterols or stanols and ω-3 fatty acids, plus antihypertensive, antidiabetic and lipid-regulating drug therapy as necessary. Statins are considered to be the mainstay of the latter and should be given to all those with CVD, diabetics over the age of 40 years and high-risk patients who fail to achieve optimal lipid levels by lifestyle changes within 3 months. Although the target level of LDL cholesterol in JBS2 (<2 mmol/L) is more radical than that in the previous Joint British Societies' guidelines, the alternative criterion of a 30% reduction appears to be anomalously small. For example, the data shown in Table 7.4 of Chapter 7 suggest that reductions in the range of 40–50% are needed to achieve LDL levels in the region of 2 mmol/L.

Prevention of cardiovascular disease in diabetes mellitus

Dyslipidaemia is now recognized to be the major risk factor for macrovascular disease in type 2 diabetics. Subgroup analysis of the 4S study showed that reduction of LDL cholesterol with simvastatin decreased the incidence of coronary and cerebrovascular events to a similar extent in diabetics as in non-diabetics, with diabetics on placebo exhibiting a markedly increased frequency of CHD events compared with non-diabetics.[29] Similar results have been observed in several other studies, including a recent primary prevention trial, which showed that atorvastatin at 10 mg daily reduced major CVD events by 37% in type 2 diabetics in the UK and Ireland.[30]

Various guidelines have been issued on this topic, including a statement from the American Heart Association,[31] which advocates a rigorous diet (Step 2) for all diabetics with recourse to lipid-lowering drug therapy if LDL cholesterol remains above 3.4 mmol/L, the target level being <3.4 mmol/L. Secondary goals of treatment are to reduce triglycerides to below 2.3 mmol/L and raise HDL cholesterol above 0.9 mmol/L. Statins are recommended as first-line drug therapy, either alone or combined with a fibrate in those with a fasting triglyceride above 4.5 mmol/L. Like JBS2, the updated version of ATP III no longer differentiates between primary and secondary prevention in diabetics, and sets optional goals for LDL cholesterol and non-HDL cholesterol of <1.8 and <2.6 mmol/L, respectively.

APPLICATION OF GUIDELINES

Despite slight differences of emphasis, all the guidelines agree that patients with CHD have the highest priority for treatment. Evidence that this advice has not always been implemented as regards dyslipidaemia comes from a UK survey of almost 2000 patients with CHD in general practice; blood pressure was managed in accordance with guidelines in 82% but serum lipids in only 17%.[32]

Similarly disappointing results were reported by Euroaspire II,[33] which surveyed more than 5000 patients with CHD at 6 months post-admission to hospital in 15 countries and compared their risk factor status with the goals of the Second Joint European Societies' guidelines.[27] Total cholesterol exceeded the recommended level of 5 mmol/L in 58% of patients, HDL cholesterol was <1 mmol/L in 23% and triglyceride was >2 mmol/L in 29%. Of the 61% of patients on a lipid-lowering drug, total cholesterol was >5 mmol/L in 50% of them. Control of smoking, blood pressure and, in diabetics, blood glucose, was also inadequate.

Barriers to implementation of therapeutic guidelines arise from three sources.[26] Those that are physician-related include lack of knowledge of guidelines and difficulty in interpreting them. The main health care barrier is budgetary restraint, whereas patient-related barriers include time constraints and poor compliance. It has been estimated that 30% of patients discontinue taking statins within 6–7 months[34] and that 50% of them stop completely after 5 years.[35] The major benefits that have been shown to accrue from effective use of statins makes it imperative to overcome these obstacles by means of better medical education of medical students at undergraduate and postgraduate levels, greater awareness of the importance of controlling risk factors among patients, and decreasing the costs of statins as their patents run out.

REFERENCES

1. Department of Health. Report on Health and Social Subjects No. 46. Nutritional aspects of cardiovascular disease. London: HMSO, 1994.
2. Report of a Joint Working Party of the Royal College of Physicians of London and the British Cardiac Society. Prevention of coronary heart disease. J Roy Coll Physicians 1976; 10:214–75.
3. Report from the Committee of Principal Investigators. A co-operative trial in the primary prevention of ischaemic heart disease using clofibrate. Br Heart J 1978; 40:1069–118.
4. Committee of Principal Investigators. WHO co-operative trial on primary prevention of ischaemic heart disease using clofibrate to lower serum cholesterol: mortality follow-up. Lancet 1980; 2:379–85.
5. Lipid Research Clinics Program. The Lipid Research Clinics Coronary Primary Prevention Trial results. 1. Reduction in incidence of coronary heart disease. J Am Med Assoc 1984; 251: 351–64.
6. Consensus Conference. Lowering blood cholesterol to prevent heart disease. J Am Med Assoc 1985; 253:2080–6.
7. Shepherd J, Betteridge DJ, Durrington P et al. Strategies for reducing coronary heart disease and desirable limits for blood lipid concentrations: guidelines of the British Hyperlipidaemia Association. Br Med J 1987; 295:1245–6.
8. Betteridge DJ, Dodson PM, Durrington PN et al. Management of hyperlipidaemia: guidelines of the British Hyperlipidaemia Association. Postgrad Med J 1993; 69:359–69.
9. European Atherosclerosis Society Study Group. Strategies for the prevention of coronary heart disease: a policy statement of the European Atherosclerosis Society. Eur Heart J 1987; 8:77–88.
10. European Atherosclerosis Society Study Group. The recognition and management of hyperlipidaemia in adults: a policy statement of the European Atherosclerosis Society. Eur Heart J 1988; 9:571–600.
11. European Atherosclerosis Society International Task Force for Prevention of Coronary Heart Disease. Prevention of coronary heart disease: scientific background and new clinical guidelines. Nutr Metab Cardiovasc Dis 1992; 2:113–56.

12. The Expert Panel. Report of the National Cholesterol Education Program Expert Panel on detection, evaluation, and treatment of high blood cholesterol in adults. Arch Int Med 1988; 148:36–69.
13. Pyörälä K, De Backer G, Graham I et al. Prevention of coronary heart disease in clinical practice. Recommendations of the Task Force of the European Society of Cardiology, European Atherosclerosis Society and European Society of Hypertension. Eur Heart J 1994; 15:1300–31.
14. Scandinavian Simvastatin Survival Study Group. Randomised trial of cholesterol lowering in 4444 patients with coronary heart disease: the Scandinavian Simvastatin Survival Study (4S). Lancet 1994; 344:1383–9.
15. Pearce ML, Dayton S. Incidence of cancer in men on a diet high in polyunsaturated fat. Lancet 1971; 1:464.
16. Oliver M. Might treatment of hypercholesterolaemia increase non-cardiac mortality? Lancet 1991; 337:1529–31.
17. Muldoon MF, Manuck SB, Matthews KA. Lowering cholesterol concentrations and mortality: a quantitative review of primary prevention trials. Br Med J 1990; 301:309–14.
18. Thompson GR. Cholesterol lowering and non-cardiac mortality. Lancet 1991; 338:126.
19. Law MR, Thompson SG, Wald NJ. Assessing possible hazards of reducing serum cholesterol. Br Med J 1994; 308:373–9.
20. Expert Panel on Detection, Evaluation and Treatment of High Cholesterol in Adults. Summary of the Second Report of the National Cholesterol Education Program (NCEP) Expert Panel on detection, evaluation, and treatment of high blood cholesterol in adults (Adult Treatment Panel II). J Am Med Assoc 1993; 269:3015–23.
21. Expert Panel on Detection, Evaluation and Treatment of High Cholesterol in Adults. Executive Summary of the Third Report of the National Cholesterol Education Program (NCEP) Expert Panel on detection, evaluation, and treatment of high blood cholesterol in adults (Adult Treatment Panel III). J Am Med Assoc 2001; 285:2486–97.
22. Heart Protection Study Collaborative Group. MRC/BHF Heart Protection Study of cholesterol lowering with simvastatin in 20536 high risk individuals: a randomised placebo-controlled trial. Lancet 2002; 360:7–22.
23. Grundy SM, Cleeman JI, Bairey Merz N et al. Implications of recent clinical trials for the National Cholesterol Education Program Adult Treatment Panel III Guidelines. Circulation 2004; 110:227–39.
24. The International Task Force for Prevention of Coronary Heart Disease/International Atherosclerosis Society. Coronary heart disease: reducing the risk. Nutr Metab Cardiovasc Dis 1998; 8:205–71.
25. Haq IU, Ramsay LE, Yeo WW, Jackson PR, Wallis EJ. Is the Framingham risk function valid for northern European populations? A comparison of methods for estimating absolute coronary risk in high risk men. Heart 1999; 81:40–6.
26. De Backer G, Abrosioni E, Borch-Johnsen K et al. European guidelines on cardiovascular disease prevention in clinical practice. Third Joint Task Force of European and other Societies on Cardiovascular Disease Prevention in Clinical Practice. Eur J Cardiovasc Prevent Rehab 2003; 10(Suppl 1):S1–S78.
27. Wood D, De Backer G, Faergeman O et al, together with members of the Task Force. Prevention of coronary heart disease in clinical practice: recommendations of the Second Joint Task Force of European and other Societies on Coronary Prevention. Atherosclerosis 1998; 140:199–270.
28. British Cardiac Society, British Hypertension Society, Diabetes UK, HEART UK, Primary Care Cardiovascular Society, The Stroke Association. JBS2: Joint British Societies' guidelines on prevention of cardiovascular disease in clinical practice. Heart 2005; 91(Suppl V): v1–v52.
29. Pyorala K, Pedersen TR, Kjekshus J et al and the Scandinavian Simvastatin Survival Study Group. Cholesterol lowering with simvastatin improves prognosis of diabetic patients with coronary heart disease. Diabetes Care 1997; 20:614–20.

30. Colhoun HM, Betteridge DJ, Durrington PN et al. Primary prevention of cardiovascular disease with atorvastatin in type 2 diabetes in the Collaborative Atorvastatin Diabetes Study (CARDS): multicentre randomised placebo-controlled trial. Lancet 2004; 364:685–96.

31. Grundy SM, Benjamin IJ, Burke GL et al. Diabetes and cardiovascular disease. A statement for healthcare professionals from the American Heart Association. Circulation 1999; 100:1134–46.

32. Campbell NC, Thain J, Deans HG et al. Secondary prevention in coronary heart disease: baseline survey of provision in general practice. Br Med J 1998; 316: 1430–4.

33. EUROASPIRE II Study Group. Lifestyle and risk factor management and use of drug therapies in coronary patients from 15 countries; principal results from EUROASPIRE II Euro Heart Survey Programme. Eur Heart J 2001; 22:526–8.

34. Simons LA, Simons J, McManus P, Dudley J. Discontinuation rates for use of statins are high. Br Med J 2000; 321: 1084.

35. Avorn J, Monette J, Lacour A et al. Persistence of use of lipid-lowering medications: a cross-national study. J Am Med Assoc 1998; 279:1458–62.

7

Pharmacological management of dyslipidaemia

INTRODUCTION

Lipid regulating drug therapy is indicated in patients with coronary heart disease (CHD) and high-risk individuals in whom dietary and lifestyle measures have failed to control dyslipidaemia. The guidelines described in Chapter 6 provide information as to when and in whom drug therapy should be embarked upon. Because this is usually a life-long commitment, the use of these drugs should be the exception rather than the rule in asymptomatic patients, being restricted to those with severe hyperlipidaemia of genetic origin, such as familial hypercholesterolaemia (FH), or in whom the presence of other risk factors results in an unacceptably high risk. The latter is commonly defined as ≥20% / 10 years for CHD events or ≥5% / 10 years for fatal CVD. The opposite applies, however, to patients with clinically manifest CHD, in whom even mild dyslipidaemia requires vigorous drug therapy aimed at achieving target levels stipulated in guidelines.

The rationale for the use of lipid regulating drugs is based on the large body of evidence from epidemiological and clinicopathological studies that points to the central role of cholesterol in atherosclerosis, as discussed in Chapter 2. Confirmation that the association is causal comes from numerous angiographic and clinical endpoint studies showing that lipid-lowering therapy slows the rate of progression of atherosclerotic lesions in coronary, carotid and femoral arteries, and reduces the frequency of associated cardiovascular events. The best proof of causality derives from the atherogenicity of low density lipoprotein (LDL) and the evidence that lowering LDL cholesterol arrests or reverses the process. Loss of the protective effect of high density lipoprotein (HDL), resulting from a decrease in plasma levels, also has strong epidemiological support, but the evidence that raising HDL cholesterol is beneficial is less compelling. Likewise, although increasing epidemiological and angiographic evidence suggests that triglyceride-rich remnant particles play a role in promoting the progression of mild-to-moderate lesions in coronary arteries, more data are needed on whether lowering triglyceride prevents CHD events. Hence, it is not surprising that the current therapeutic emphasis is on lowering LDL cholesterol. That said, there is increasing interest in developing compounds that raise HDL cholesterol and could be used as an adjunct to LDL-lowering drugs.

LIPID REGULATING DRUGS

The effects of the various classes of drugs used to modulate serum lipid levels are shown in Table 7.1. Hydroxymethyl glutaryl coenzyme A (HMGCoA) reductase inhibitors or statins, exemplified by atorvastatin, are the most potent means of reducing LDL cholesterol and, in addition, they reduce triglyceride and cause a modest increase in HDL cholesterol. Bile acid sequestrants, exemplified by colestyramine, are a moderately effective means of reducing LDL cholesterol and increasing HDL cholesterol, but they cause a potentially undesirable increase in serum triglyceride. Ezetimide, a recently introduced cholesterol absorption inhibitor, has similar efficacy in lowering LDL but little effect on HDL cholesterol or triglyceride. Nicotinic acid and its analogues are the most effective means of increasing HDL cholesterol and also have a useful triglyceride-lowering effect. Fibric acid derivatives, exemplified by gemfibrozil, are the most effective means of reducing triglyceride and also have a modest HDL cholesterol-raising effect. The commonly used doses, indications and side-effects of the main lipid regulating drugs in current use are summarized in Table 7.2. More detailed descriptions of each class of drugs and of individual compounds are given below.

Fibric acid derivatives

Of the three main classes of lipid-lowering drugs, the longest established are the fibrates, which promote lipolysis by stimulating lipoprotein lipase via their interaction with PPAR*α and -γ in the liver and adipose tissue, respectively.[1]

The five compounds marketed in the UK are clofibrate, bezafibrate, fenofibrate, gemfibrozil and ciprofibrate. All are effective in controlling hypertriglyceridaemia and in raising HDL cholesterol, but their ability to reduce LDL cholesterol is relatively modest, fenofibrate and ciprofibate being the most potent. Clofibrate, the prototype, has been in use for over 30 years but is now obsolete. Its main action is to stimulate chylomicron and very low density lipoprotein (VLDL) lipolysis by

Table 7.1   Comparative effects of lipid regulating drugs

Daily dose	Mean change (%)		
	LDL-C	HDL-C	TG
Atorvastatin 40 mg	−51	+5	−32
Nicotinic acid 4 g	−9	+43	−34
Gemfibrozil 1.2 g	−18	+12	−40
Ezetimibe 10 mg	−18.5	+3.5	−4.9
Colestyramine 24 g	−23	+8	+11

TC, total cholesterol; LDL-C, low density lipoprotein cholesterol; HDL-C, high density lipoprotein cholesterol; TG, triglyceride.

* Peroxisome proliferator activated receptor; see also Chapter 1.

	Indications	Side-effects	Contraindications
s .d.	Hypercholesterolaemia	Gastrointestinal dysfunction	Hypertriglyceridaemia peptic ulcer, haemorrh
o.d. o.d. b.d. o.d.	Hypertriglyceridaemia, mixed hyperlipidaemia	Myositis-like syndrome, increased bile lithogenicity, pruritis, urticaria, impotence, headache, vertigo, dizziness, fatigue, hair loss	Renal or hepatic impai gall bladder disease, pregnancy, breast-feed cirrhosis
inhibitors g o.d. g o.d. g b.d. g o.d. mg o.d. mg o.d.	Hypercholesterolaemia, mixed hyperlipidaemia	Hepatic dysfunction, myositis, rhabdomyolysis, gastrointestinal disturbances, headache, fatigue, insomnia	Liver disease, cyclospo therapy, pregnancy, br feeding
alogues d.s.	Hypertriglyceridaemia	Gastrointestinal disturbances, vasodilatation, flushing, rash, itching, headaches.	Pregnancy, breast-feedi peptic ulcer (acipimox). Caution in patients wit gout, diabetes, liver dis
	Severe hypertriglyceridaemia	Nausea, odour, can raise LDL	Hypercholesterolaemia
inhibitors .	Hypercholesterolaemia	Gastrointestinal disturbances, headache, rash	Hepatic dysfunction, breast-feeding

increasing adipose tissue-derived lipoprotein lipase. Daily doses of 0.5–1.0 g b.d., result in a 15–20% decrease in serum total cholesterol and a 30–40% decrease in serum triglyceride, but in hypertriglyceridaemic patients this often leads to an undesirable increase in LDL cholesterol. Patients with type III hyperlipoproteinaemia usually respond dramatically, with virtual normalization of serum lipids and regression of cutaneous xanthomas.

Administration of clofibrate increases biliary cholesterol secretion, which increases the risk of developing gallstones by twofold. The other major side-effect of clofibrate and of other fibrates is an acute myositic syndrome characterized by pain in the thighs or calves and by an increase in creatine phosphokinase (CPK). Patients with renal impairment are particularly vulnerable.

Bezafibrate decreases levels of VLDL more effectively than clofibrate in hypertriglyceridaemia, but there is little difference between them in lowering LDL cholesterol and raising HDL cholesterol levels in individuals with hypercholesterolaemia or mixed hyperlipidaemia. As with clofibrate, a significant rise in LDL cholesterol has been observed in hypertriglyceridaemic patients during treatment.

Gemfibrozil is a homologue of clofibrate but has a much shorter plasma half-life. Its mechanism of action is similar, although it decreases LDL cholesterol to a lesser extent than bezafibrate and appears to be less lithogenic than clofibrate, as judged from the results of the Helsinki Heart Study. During that trial, the average changes in serum lipids induced by gemfibrozil 1.2 g daily were an 11% decrease in total cholesterol, 10% decrease in LDL cholesterol, 43% decrease in triglyceride and a 10% increase in HDL cholesterol.[2]

Fenofibrate has a slightly longer half-life in plasma than clofibrate but is six times more potent on a weight basis and has a significant hypo-uricaemic effect. Ciprofibrate has the longest plasma half-life of all the fibric acid derivatives, which may account for its reputedly greater myotoxicity.

Clinical outcome trials

Two primary prevention trials, the WHO trial of clofibrate[3] and the Helsinki Heart Study of gemfibrozil[4] provided evidence that fibrates have the ability to reduce the incidence of CHD in patients with moderate hypercholesterolaemia, although with clofibrate this was offset by an increased incidence of non-cardiac causes of death.[5]

Statistical analysis of the Helsinki Heart Study suggested that the beneficial effects of gemfibrozil were due partly to the reduction in LDL cholesterol and partly to the increase in HDL cholesterol. Benefit was most marked in a subgroup of individuals with triglyceride >2.3 mmol/L and LDL:HDL cholesterol ratio >5.[6] Additional evidence of the benefits of gemfibrozil came from the Veterans Affairs High Density Lipoprotein Cholesterol Intervention Trial (VAHIT), which showed that the drug reduced the risk of further events in elderly men with CHD and a low HDL cholesterol.[7]

The Bezafibrate Infarction Prevention (BIP) trial demonstrated the benefit of bezafibrate in secondary prevention, although this was restricted to a subgroup of volunteers with raised serum triglyceride.[8] An international consensus on the therapeutic role of fibrates has been published.[9]

Bile acid sequestrants

The bile acid sequestrants (anion-exchange resins) are insoluble compounds which act by binding bile acids within the intestinal lumen, thus interfering with their reabsorption and enhancing their faecal excretion. As a result, bile acid synthesis is markedly stimulated, the increased requirement for cholesterol in the liver being met partly by up-regulation of hepatic LDL receptors. The advantage resins have in being unabsorbed is offset, however, by their unappetising consistency and bulk and high frequency of gastrointestinal side-effects, which decrease compliance.

Colestyramine (previously spelt cholestyramine) has been in use for almost 30 years. In the Lipid Research Clinics Coronary Primary Prevention Trial (CPPT), men with moderate hypercholesterolaemia were prescribed colestyramine at 24 g daily. Over a period of seven years their mean total cholesterol was 8.5% lower, LDL cholesterol 12.6% lower, HDL cholesterol 3% higher and triglyceride 4.5% higher than placebo-treated controls.[10] Much greater reductions in LDL cholesterol (26–33%) were observed in patients known to be taking at least 20 grams of the drug per day, but almost 30% of patients discontinued taking it before the end of the trial.[11]

The most frequent side-effects are constipation, which occasionally leads to intestinal obstruction, and a tendency to aggravate or cause indigestion. Colestyramine also engenders an increase in VLDL synthesis, making it unsuitable for treating patients with hypertriglyceridaemia.

Colestipol hydrochloride is less widely used than colestyramine but has a similar mode of action. The usual daily dose is 10 g b.d. There is little to choose between colestyramine and colestipol with regard to extent of LDL cholesterol-lowering and side-effects. Interference with the absorption of iron and folic acid necessitates their provision as supplements in the diets of children who have been treated with resins.

Clinical outcome trials

Colestyramine treated volunteers in the CPPT sustained a 19% reduction in CHD deaths and non-fatal myocardial infarcts ($P < 0.05$) compared with those on placebo but no decrease in total mortality.[10] The extent of benefit depended upon the reduction in serum cholesterol achieved, which reflected drug compliance.[11] This trial demonstrated for the first time the importance of reducing LDL cholesterol and was the forerunner of the statin trials, which achieved much greater reductions in LDL.

HMG CoA reductase inhibitors

This class of drug acts by competitively inhibiting HMG CoA reductase and thereby blocking conversion of HMG CoA to mevalonic acid. As a result, cholesterol synthesis is inhibited, especially in the liver which requires cholesterol as a substrate for bile acid synthesis. This leads to an increased expression of hepatic LDL receptors and greater uptake of LDL cholesterol from plasma. Production of LDL is also decreased, the net effect being a dose-dependent reduction in LDL cholesterol of up to 60%, accompanied by a lesser reduction in plasma triglyceride and a small rise in HDL cholesterol (Table 7.1).

The HMG CoA reductase inhibitors have a similar spectrum of action to the bile acid sequestrants in that they mainly lower LDL cholesterol, but they also reduce serum triglyceride, unlike resins, which show the opposite tendency. HMG CoA

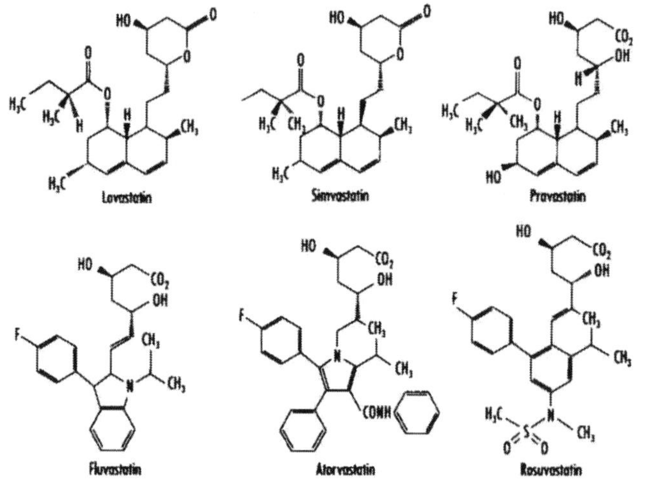

Figure 7.1   Structure of the six statins in common use.

reductase inhibitors are more effective than bile acid sequestrants in lowering LDL cholesterol, but less effective than the fibrates in reducing serum triglyceride and in raising HDL cholesterol.

The chemical formulas of the six statins marketed in most parts of the world are shown in Figure 7.1. The first HMGCoA reductase inhibitor to be developed and licensed in the USA, but not the UK, was lovastatin, which is a fungal metabolite. Simvastatin is a methylated derivative of lovastatin whereas pravastatin is made from a different mould. Fluvastatin, the first HMGCoA reductase inhibitor to be produced synthetically, is a racemate whereas the other two synthetic compounds, atorvastatin and rosuvastatin, are both active enantiomers.

The fungal derivatives are all structurally similar, but lovastatin and simvastatin are administered as lactones, which undergo conversion into the biologically-active open acid after absorption, whereas pravastatin and the synthetic statins are all administered as active compounds. Other differences are that lovastatin and simvastatin and their metabolites are more lipophilic than pravastatin, which is less completely protein-bound in plasma than other statins. First-pass uptake by the liver is high, but, despite decreasing cholesterol synthesis, these drugs do not impair the synthesis of adrenocortical and gonadal hormones, although they may decrease the formation of intermediate products of HMGCoA reductase, such as ubiquinone and dolichol.

Dose efficacy

Until recently, atorvastatin was the most effective statin available, decreasing LDL cholesterol by 41–61% when given to hypercholesterolaemic patients in doses of 10–80 mg daily.[12] Furthermore, the highest dose was shown to decrease serum triglyceride by 45% in individuals with hypertriglyceridaemia. However, rosuvastatin, which was launched subsequently, is even more effective than atorvastatin in lowering LDL cholesterol over its licensed dose range of 10–40 mg (Figure 7.2),[13]

Table 7.3   Comparative effects of statins on serum lipids[15]

Dose 40 mg/day	% change		
	LDL-C	TG	HDL-C
Atorvastatin	−50	−29	+6
Fluvastatin	−24	−10	+8
Lovastatin	−34	−24	+9
Pravastatin	−34	−24	+12
Rosuvastatin	−63	−28	+10
Simvastatin	−41	−18	+12

For abbreviations see Table 7.1.

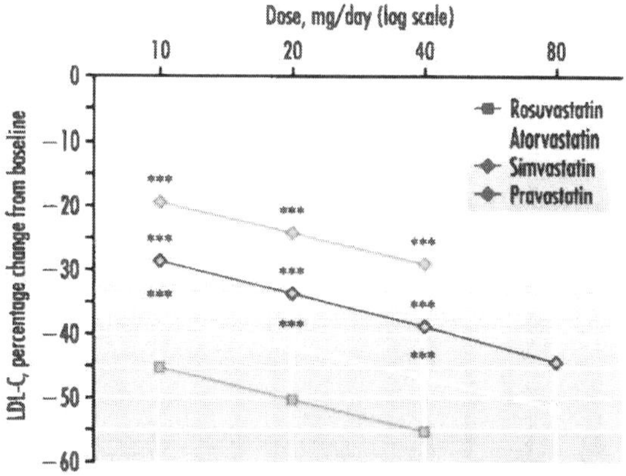

Figure 7.2   Cholesterol-lowering efficacy of rosuvastatin versus atorvastatin, simvastatin and pravastatin (reproduced with permission from the BMJ publishing group, Heart 2004; 90: 949–55).[13] ***$P < 0.001$ vs rosuvastatin at same dose. LDL-C, low density lipoprotein cholesterol.

although there was no significant difference between rosuvastatin at 40 mg and atorvastatin at 80 mg in this respect.[14] A comparison of the effects of equal doses of all the statins on serum lipids is shown in Table 7.3.[15]

The greater LDL-lowering efficacy of rosuvastatin and atorvastatin compared with other statins reflects the longer residence time of these drugs or their active metabolites in the liver, resulting in more prolonged inhibition of HMG CoA reductase and decreased secretion of apoB-containing lipoproteins; the latter action explains their ability to lower both serum cholesterol and triglyceride. Compared with fenofibrate, atorvastatin at 10–20 mg daily was more effective in lowering LDL cholesterol in patients with combined hyperlipidaemia but less effective in decreasing triglyceride and in raising HDL cholesterol.[16] However, the non-HDL:HDL cholesterol ratio was lower in those on atorvastatin than on fenofibrate, reflecting the greater decrease in LDL.

The ultimate test for any cholesterol-lowering agent is homozygous FH, which is refractory to most drugs and usually necessitates the use of radical measures such as apheresis or liver transplantation. In such individuals, atorvastatin at 80 mg daily achieved a 31% decrease in LDL cholesterol, mainly by reducing the rate of LDL production.[17] As might be expected, a greater decrease in LDL cholesterol, averaging 57%, was observed in FH heterozygotes,[18] in whom deficiency of LDL receptors is less marked than in homozygotes.

Safety

The largest and most carefully controlled assessment of safety was the Expanded Clinical Evaluation of Lovastatin (EXCEL) study, in which 8245 patients received placebo or lovastatin, 20–80 mg daily for 48 weeks.[19] This showed asymptomatic and reversible increases in hepatic transaminases in approximately 2% of individuals, which were dose related and usually resolved if the drug was withdrawn or its dosage reduced. A similar pattern is seen with other statins.

The most important adverse effect of statins is myositis, defined as muscle pain plus an increase in creatine phosphokinase (CPK) greater than ten times the upper limit of normal. Rarely, severe rhabdomyolysis leading to fatal renal damage has occurred, and the synthetic HMG CoA reductase inhibitor, cerivastatin, was withdrawn recently on this account. Other statins have a remarkably good safety record: an analysis of data from over 30 000 patients who had received pravastatin, simvastatin or lovastatin for a period of 5 years or more found that the incidence of myositis was only 0.1%, identical to that on placebo. In the Heart Protection Study the frequency of CPK elevations greater than ten times the upper limit of normal was 0.09% in patients on simvastatin compared with 0.05% in those on placebo.[20] The likelihood of this complication occurring is dose related and is increased by concomitant treatment with drugs such as cyclosporine, which inhibit the cytochrome P450 3A4 pathway via which several statins are metabolized.[15]

Clinical outcome trials

Evidence of a reduction in cardiovascular events during statin therapy has come from three secondary prevention trials using (i) simvastatin (Scandinavian Simvastatin Survival Study [4S][21]), (ii) pravastatin (Cholesterol and Recurrent Events [CARE][22]) and (iii) provastatin (Long-Term Intervention with Pravastatin in Ischaemic Disease [LIPID][23]). Two primary prevention trials have involved pravastatin (West of Scotland Coronary Prevention Study [WOSCOPS][24]) and lovastatin (Air Force/Texas Coronary Atherosclerosis Prevention Study [AF/TexCAPS][25]). Overall, statins reduced total and LDL cholesterol by 20% and 28%, respectively, and decreased the risk of CHD by 31% and total mortality by 21%; these benefits were equally evident in men and women and below and above the age of 65 years.[26]

As well as a decreased incidence of myocardial infarction and reduced need for re-vascularization procedures, a significant decrease in stroke was apparent on post-hoc analysis of the results of the 4S study and was also evident in the CARE and LIPID studies, where it was a pre-determined end-point. A meta-analysis of the results of these and other trials using simvastatin, lovastatin or pravastatin, involving almost 10 000 patients, showed a 27% decrease in the risk of stroke.[27]

Other cardiovascular effects of statins include a reduced frequency of Holter-monitored episodes of myocardial ischaemia, presumably by improving vascular endothelial function. The latter probably reflects the LDL-lowering effect of statins in that endothelial function is inversely correlated with the level of LDL cholesterol and improves also when LDL is lowered by other means. Whether the anti-inflammatory effects of statins are LDL-dependent is more debatable, since they are evident in atheromatous plaques within a month of starting treatment.[28] Either mechanism could explain the beneficial effects of starting statin therapy within the first few days after the onset of an acute coronary syndrome.[29]

How low should LDL go?

The extent to which LDL cholesterol should be reduced by treatment is uncertain but evidence from four recent statin trials supports the concept 'the lower the better'. In the Atorvastatin Versus Revascularization Treatment (AVERT) Trial patients with stable angina treated with atorvastatin at 80 mg daily had fewer ischaemic events than those who underwent angioplasty and received usual care.[30] The results of the Reversal of Atherosclerosis with Aggressive Lipid Lowering (REVERSAL) and the Pravastatin or Atorvastatin Evaluation and Infection Therapy-Thrombolysis in Myocardial Infarction 22 (PROVE IT-TIMI 22) trials[31,32] showed that atorvastatin at 80 mg daily was of greater benefit in preventing progression of coronary atherosclerosis and reducing cardiovascular events, respectively, than was pravastatin at 40 mg daily. In the most recent trial, the Treating to New Targets (TNT) investigators showed that fewer cardiovascular events occurred on atorvastatin at 80 mg than at 10 mg daily, although there was a sixfold increase in raised transaminase levels at the higher dose.[33] As shown in Table 7.4, patients on a daily dose of 80 mg atorvastatin in these four trials had LDL cholesterol levels averaging ≤2 mmol/L, with reductions of 42–49%, while those on usual care or lower doses of statins had LDL cholesterol levels ranging from 2.5–3 mmol/L and reductions of 10–33%.

In the meta-analysis of statin trials performed by the Antihypertensive and Lipid-Lowering Treatment to Prevent Heart Attack Trial (ALLHAT) investigators,[34] extrapolation of the regression line correlating the log odds ratio for CHD events

Table 7.4 Comparison of LDL-lowering effects of atorvastatin given at 80 mg daily versus usual care or lower doses of atorvastatin or pravastatin in four recent intervention trials.[33-35]

Trial	Treatment groups	On treatment	
		LDL-C (mmol/L)	Δ% LDL-C
AVERT	PTCA and usual care	3.0	18%
	Atorvastatin 80 mg	2.0	46%
REVERSAL	Pravastatin 40 mg	2.8	27%
	Atorvastatin 80 mg	2.0	47%
PROVE IT-TIMI 22	Pravastatin 40 mg	2.5	10%
	Atorvastatin 80 mg	1.6	42%
TNT	Atorvastatin 10 mg	2.6	33%
	Atorvastatin 80 mg	2.0	49%

PTCA, percutaneous transluminal coronary angioplasty

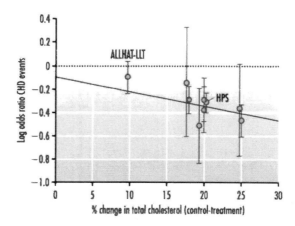

Figure 7.3 Reductions in coronary heart disease (CHD) in cholesterol-lowering trials, including the lipid-lowering trial component of the Anti-hypertensive and Lipid-Lowering Treatment to Prevent Heart Attack Trial (ALLHAT-LLT) and The Heart Protection Study (HPS). (Reproduced with permission from Ref 34.)

with the percentage change in total cholesterol (Figure 7.3) suggests that a decrease in total cholesterol of 36%, equivalent to a decrease in LDL cholesterol of 50%, would halve the risk of CHD. Reductions in LDL cholesterol of this magnitude are perfectly feasible using maximum doses of atorvastatin and rosuvastatin alone, or of simvastatin combined with ezetimibe, as discussed later.

Role of C-reactive protein

Clinical outcome in two of the four trials which compared high versus lower dose statin therapy was related not only to the LDL cholesterol level on treatment, but also to the extent of reduction of C-reactive protein (CRP). It is debatable whether CRP is a risk factor in its own right or simply an inflammatory marker. Analysis of the results of PROVE IT-TIMI 22 showed that coronary events were lowest in patients with LDL cholesterol <1.8 mmol/L and CRP <2 mg/l and highest in those with LDL >1.8 mmol/L and CRP >2 mg/l.[35] Intermediate but similar event rates were observed in those with LDL cholesterol <1.8 mmol/L and CRP >2 mg/l or with LDL cholesterol >1.8 mmol/L and CRP <2 mg/l. Analogous findings occurred in the REVERSAL trial, where the rate of progression of coronary lesions was significantly correlated with the decrease in CRP levels, progression being slowest in patients with the greatest reductions in both LDL cholesterol and CRP.[36] In both trials CRP and LDL decreases were significantly but only weakly correlated, indicating that the former was not simply a consequence of the latter. This raises the question of how one should manage patients in whom maximal statin therapy lowers LDL cholesterol to the requisite target level but whose CRP remains high. Answers to this and other questions are needed before measurement of CRP can be regarded as an integral part of coronary risk assessment and therapeutic decision-making.

OTHER LIPID REGULATING COMPOUNDS

Nicotinic acid

The lipid regulating effect of large doses of nicotinic acid was first described in 1962. Long-term follow-up of patients who participated in the Coronary Drug Project showed a reduction in mortality in those who had taken nicotinic acid during the trial. The drug would be more widely used were it not for its side-effects, which include cutaneous flushing, skin rashes, gastrointestinal upsets, hyperuricaemia, hyperglycaemia and hepatic dysfunction. Sustained release preparations reduce flushing but accentuate the risk of hepatitis.

Recently an extended-release form of nicotinic acid (Niaspan) has been developed, which seems to be free from this drawback. At the maximum recommended dose of 2 g daily, decreases in LDL cholesterol, triglyceride and Lp(a) averaged 17%, 35% and 24%, respectively, whereas HDL cholesterol increased by 26%. Although 30% of those randomized to Niaspan had troublesome side-effects, the frequency of abnormal liver function tests was similar to that on placebo.[37]

Ezetimibe

Recently, it was shown that a specific protein (NPC1L1) mediates the uptake of cholesterol from the lumen into the wall of the small intestine (see Chapter 1). A novel class of compounds, 2-azetidinone derivatives, has now been shown to interact with this cholesterol transporter in the intestinal brush border membrane, thereby inhibiting cholesterol and plant sterol absorption. The first of these cholesterol absorption inhibitors to be licensed is ezetimibe.

Randomized, placebo controlled trials of ezetimibe in hypercholesterolaemic patients show dose-dependent reductions in LDL cholesterol over the range 0.25–10 mg daily. The mean decrease in LDL cholesterol on 10 mg daily was 18.2%, which was accompanied by small but significant increases in HDL cholesterol and decreases in serum triglyceride.[38] The drug was well tolerated and the frequency of adverse events was similar to that in the placebo group. Because its LDL-lowering ability is only moderate, its main use is likely to be as an adjunct to statin therapy.

ω-3 fatty acids

The diet contains ω-3 fatty acids as long chain, polyunsaturated triglyceride derived from plant and marine sources. The three main compounds are α-linolenic acid (ALA or 18:3ω-3), eicosapentaenoic acid (EPA or 20:5ω-3) and docosahexaenoic acid (DHA or 22:5ω-3). ALA is mainly derived from vegetable oils, EPA and DHA from oily fish. Capsules of fish oil (Maxepa) or ethyl esters of EPA and DHA (Omacor) are licensed for prescription in the UK.

In the light of the apparent protection from CHD observed initially in Eskimos, several prospective studies examined the relationship between ω-3 fatty acids and CHD in other populations. The results were inconclusive but suggested a possible protective effect against sudden death from CHD, emphasizing the need for randomized controlled clinical trials. A subsequent meta-analysis of the results of 11 such trials showed that the risk of fatal myocardial infarction was reduced by 30% ($P < 0.001$) and total mortality by 20% ($P < 0.001$) in those receiving ω-3 fatty acids.[39]

Triglyceride decreased by an average of 20% but little change was observed in LDL or HDL cholesterol.

Data from several sources suggest that ω-3 fatty acids protect against sudden death from CHD rather than non-fatal events. Experimental evidence in animals suggests an anti-arrhythmic mechanism of action of EPA and DHA, but more data are needed to substantiate this in humans. The dose of ω-3 fatty acids for secondary prevention is 1 g daily, equivalent to 100 g of oily fish, whereas higher doses (2–4 g daily) of EPA and DHA are used to treat severe hypertriglyceridaemia.

COMBINATION THERAPY

Monotherapy with statins does not always lower LDL cholesterol and triglyceride or raise HDL cholesterol to the required extent and it may be necessary to combine their administration with other lipid regulating drugs. For example, in severe FH even maximal doses of statins may fail to lower LDL cholesterol sufficiently and an anion-exchange resin is often added. Similarly, in mixed hyperlipidaemia, statin monotherapy may fail to reduce triglyceride and raise HDL cholesterol to the desired levels, and it may be necessary to add either nicotinic acid or a fibrate to achieve these objectives.

Another reason for combination therapy is to improve the response of patients who do not have FH but are refractory to statins. Inter-individual variability in response to these drugs is well recognized and it seems that genetic variation in cholesterol absorption efficiency is an important determinant of statin responsiveness. This was exemplified by the subgroup analysis conducted on the Finnish cohort of the 4S study, which showed that those who absorbed cholesterol efficiently and whose basal cholesterol synthesis rate was low had a lesser response to simvastatin than those whose synthesis rate was initially high.[40] Combining statins with ezetimibe, which blocks cholesterol absorption and up-regulates its synthesis, has obvious therapeutic potential in these circumstances.

Combined therapy with statins and nicotinic acid or a fibrate

The few studies which have compared statins alone and in combination with nicotinic acid or a fibrate suggest that both drugs are useful adjuncts to statins, the choice depending more on safety and tolerability than on efficacy. In hypercholesterolaemia, addition of nicotinic acid provides a greater reduction in LDL cholesterol than do fibrates and a similar increase in HDL cholesterol as statins alone. In hypertriglyceridaemia, the addition of nicotinic acid to a statin markedly reduces triglyceride and raises HDL cholesterol, whereas in mixed hyperlipidaemia the addition of a fibrate to a statin has beneficial effects on triglyceride and HDL cholesterol but at the expense of a slight increase in LDL cholesterol.

Mixed dyslipidaemia is especially common in type 2 diabetes and is a more important determinant of prognosis than is hyperglycaemia. Statins are recommended as first-line drug therapy in diabetics, either alone or combined with a fibrate, if fasting triglyceride is >4.5 mmol/L. The safety of combined statin/fibrate therapy has been questioned because of the perception that this may increase the risk of myositis. However, most of the reported cases developing this complication had received a statin combined with gemfibrozil. Other fibrates do not carry the same risk, and the chances of developing myositis with any of the statins combined with bezafibrate or fenofibrate are acceptably low.

Combined therapy with ezetimibe and statins

A study in hypercholesterolaemic patients showed that concomitant administration of ezetimibe at 10 mg and simvastatin at 10–80 mg daily decreased LDL cholesterol by 14%, triglyceride by 8% and increased HDL cholesterol by 2% more than did simvastatin alone.[41] These data suggest an additive effect of the two drugs. Further evidence of this has come from a study of 50 patients with homozgyous FH, half of whom were undergoing LDL apheresis.[42] The results showed that combined therapy with ezetimibe at 10 mg plus atorvastatin or simvastatin at 80 mg daily lowered LDL cholesterol levels by 20.5% more than statin alone. In a recent meta-analysis ezetimibe at 10 mg plus simvastatin at 80 mg lowered LDL cholesterol by 60%, an effect equivalent to that of rosuvastatin given at 40 mg daily.[43]

As with hypertension, the trend towards combination therapy in dyslipidaemia has resulted in the development of formulations containing two lipid-lowering drugs. One such formulation is the combination of ezetimibe 10 mg with simvastatin 10, 20, 40 or 80 mg (marketed as Vytorin in the USA, Inegy in the UK). The ezetimibe 10 mg combined with simvastatin 40 or 80 mg formulations are claimed to be safer and more effective than atorvastatin given at 40 and 80 mg, respectively,[44] but it remains to be seen whether ezetimibe will be used more as a means of maximizing LDL reduction with statins or of minimizing their dosage in statin-intolerant persons.

CHOICE OF DRUG

The choice of drug or drug combination is determined by various factors, foremost among which is the type of dyslipidaemia to be treated. Other considerations include evidence of benefit from treatment with the drug concerned, cost, side-effects and contraindications, such as avoidance in children or fertile women.

Recommendations for the choice of drugs in high-risk individuals whose dyslipidaemia is unresponsive to lifestyle measures are shown in Table 7.5. Statins are the first choice in hypercholesterolaemia, with the addition of ezetimibe, a bile acid sequestrant or nicotinic acid in refractory cases. Fibrates are the first choice in hyper-triglyceridaemia, with the addition of nicotinic acid or ω-3 fatty acids if necessary. Statins are the first choice in mixed hyperlipidaemia, with addition of a fibrate if raised triglyceride persists or HDL cholesterol remains low. Statins are also the first choice in individuals with low HDL cholesterol, because they both lower LDL

Table 7.5 Recommendations for drug therapy of dyslipidaemia (modified from Ref 13)

Type	First choice	If refractory
Hypercholesterolaemia	Statin	Add cholesterol absorption inhibitor, bile acid sequestrant or nicotinic acid
Hypertriglyceridaemia	Fibrate	Add nicotinic acid or ω-3 fatty acids
Mixed hyperlipidaemia	Statin	Add fibrate (not gemfibrozil)
Low HDL cholesterol	Statin	Add fibrate or nicotinic acid

Check liver function before and after 1 month on statin. Check serum creatine kinase (CK) if myalgia occurs during statin or fibrate therapy.

cholesterol and increase HDL cholesterol,[45] but addition of a fibrate or nicotinic acid may be necessary if the total : HDL cholesterol ratio remains above 5.

FUTURE DEVELOPMENTS

A number of novel compounds are currently undergoing clinical testing, including squalene synthase inhibitors, bile acid sequestrants and ileal bile acid transporter inhibitors, all of which primarily lower LDL cholesterol. So too do MTP inhibitors, which block secretion of apoB-containing lipoproteins by the small intestine and the liver, but carry the risk of causing malabsorption and fatty liver. HDL-raising compounds include PPARα agonists and cholesterol ester transfer protein inhibitors such as torcetrapib. This compound has been shown to increase HDL cholesterol by 46% when given alone and by 61% when given in conjunction with atorvastatin, the combination also resulting in an additional 17% decrease in LDL cholesterol.[46] If torcetrapib is shown to be beneficial in clinical trials, then the eventual introduction of this and similar compounds should enable patients with low HDL levels to be managed more effectively than at present.

REFERENCES

1. Staels B, Koenig W, Habib A et al. Activation of human aortic smooth-muscle cells is inhibited by PPARα but not by PPARγ activators. Nature 1998; 393:790–2.
2. Manninen V, Elo MO, Frick MH et al. Lipid alterations and decline in the incidence of coronary heart disease in the Helsinki Heart Study. J Am Med Assoc 1988; 260:641–51.
3. Report from the Committee of Principal Investigators. A co-operative trial in the primary prevention of ischaemic heart disease using clofibrate. Br Heart J 1978; 40:1069–118.
4. Frick MH, Elo O, Haapa K et al. Helsinki Heart Study: primary prevention trial with gemfibrozil in middle-aged men with dyslipidaemia. N Engl J Med 1987; 317:1237–45.
5. Committee of Principal Investigators. WHO co-operative trial on primary prevention of ischaemic heart disease using clofibrate to lower serum cholesterol: mortality follow-up. Lancet 1980; 2:379–85.
6. Manninen V, Tenkanen L, Koskinen P et al. Joint effects of serum triglyceride and LDL cholesterol and HDL cholesterol concentrations on coronary heart disease risk in the Helsinki Heart Study. Circulation 1992; 85:37–45.
7. Rubins HB, Robins SJ, Collins D et al. for the Veterans Affairs High Density Lipoprotein Cholesterol Intervention Trial Study Group. Gemfibrozil for the secondary prevention of coronary heart disease in men with low levels of high density lipoprotein cholesterol. N Engl J Med 1999; 341:410–18.
8. Israeli Society for Prevention of Heart Attacks. Secondary prevention by raising HDL cholesterol and reducing triglycerides in patients with coronary artery disease: the Bezafibrate Infarction Prevention (BIP) study. Circulation 2000; 102:21–7.
9. Fruchart JC, Brewer HB Jr, Leitersdorf E. Consensus for the use of fibrates in the treatment of dyslipoproteinemia and coronary heart disease. Am J Cardiol 1998; 81:912–17.
10. Lipid Research Clinics Program. The Lipid Research Clinics Coronary Primary Prevention Trial results. I. Reduction in incidence of coronary heart disease. J Am Med Assoc 1984; 251: 351–64.
11. Lipid Research Clinics Program. The Lipid Research Clinics Coronary Primary Prevention Trial results. II. The relationship of reduction in incidence of coronary heart disease to cholesterol lowering. J Am Med Assoc 1984; 251: 365–74.
12. Nawrocki JW, Weiss SR, Davidson MH et al. Reduction of LDL cholesterol by 25% to 60%

in patients with primary hypercholesterolemia by atorvastatin, a new HMG-CoA reductase inhibitor. Arterioscler Thromb Vasc Biol 1995; 15: 678–82.

13. Thompson GR. Management of dyslipidaemia. Heart 2004; 90:949–55.
14. Jones PH, Davidson MH, Stein, EA et al. Comparison of the efficacy and safety of rosuvastatin versus atorvastatin, simvastatin and pravastatin across doses (STELLAR trial). Am J Cardiol 2003; 92:152–60.
15. Schachter M. Chemical, pharmacokinetic and pharmacodynamic properties of statins: an update. Fund Clin Pharmacol 2004; 19:117–25.
16. Ooi TC, Heinonen T, Alaupovic P et al. Efficacy and safety of a new hydroxy-methylglutaryl-coenzyme A reductase inhibitor, atorvastatin, in patients with combined hyperlipidaemia: comparison with fenofibrate. Arterioscler Thromb Vasc Biol 1997; 17:1793–9.
17. Marais AD, Naoumova RP, Firth JC et al. Decreased production of low density lipoprotein by atorvastatin after apheresis in homozygous familial hypercholesterolemia. J Lipid Res 1997; 38:2071–8.
18. Marais AD, Firth JC, Bateman ME et al. Atorvastatin: an effective lipid-modifying agent in familial hypercholesterolemia. Arterioscler Thromb Vasc Biol 1997; 17:1527–31.
19. Bradford RH, Shear CL, Chremos AN et al. Expanded Clinical Evaluation of Lovastatin (EXCEL) study results. I. Efficacy in modifying plasma lipoproteins and adverse event profile in 8245 patients with moderate hypercholesterolemia. Arch Int Med 1991; 151:43–9.
20. Heart Protection Study Collaborative Group. MRC/BHF Heart Protection Study of cholesterol lowering with simvastatin in 20536 high-risk individuals; a randomised placebo-controlled trial. Lancet 2002; 360:7–22.
21. Scandinavian Simvastatin Survival Study Group. Randomised trial of cholesterol lowering in 4444 patients with coronary heart disease: the Scandinavian Simvastatin Survival Study (4S). Lancet 1994; 344:1383–9.
22. Sacks FM, Pfeffer MA, Moye LA et al. The effect of pravastatin on coronary events after myocardial infarction in patients with average cholesterol levels. N Engl J Med 1996; 335:1001–9.
23. The Long-Term Intervention with Pravastatin in Ischaemic Disease (LIPID) Study Group. Prevention of cardiovascular events and death with pravastatin in patients with coronary heart disease and a broad range of initial cholesterol levels. N Engl J Med 1998; 339:1349–57.
24. Shepherd J, Cobbe SM, Ford I et al. Prevention of coronary heart disease with pravastatin in men with hypercholesterolemia. West of Scotland Coronary Prevention Study Group. N Engl J Med 1995; 333:1301–7.
25. Downs JR, Clearfield M, Weis S et al. for the AFCAPS/TexCAPS Research Group. Primary prevention of acute coronary events with lovastatin in men and women with average cholesterol levels. J Am Med Assoc 1998; 279:1615–22.
26. LaRosa JC, He J, Vupputuri S. Effect of statins on risk of coronary disease: a meta-analysis of randomised controlled trials. J Am Med Assoc 1999; 282:2340–6.
27. Crouse JR III, Byington RP, Hoen HM et al. Reductase inhibitor monotherapy and stroke prevention. Arch Int Med 1997; 157:1305–10.
28. Martin-Ventura JL, Blanco-Colio LM, Gomez-Hernandez A et al. Intensive treatment with atorvastatin reduces inflammation in mononuclear cells and human atherosclerotic lesions in one month. Stroke 2005; 36:1796–1800.
29. Schwartz GG, Olsson AG, Ezekowitz MD et al. Effects of atorvastatin on early recurrent ischemic events in acute coronary syndromes: the MIRACL study: a randomized controlled trial. J Am Med Assoc 2001; 285:1711–18.
30. Pitt B, Waters D, Brown WV et al. for The Atorvastatin versus Revascularization Treatment Investigators. Aggressive lipid-lowering therapy compared with angioplasty in stable coronary artery disease. N Engl J Med 1999; 341:70–6.
31. Nissen SE, Tuzeu EM, Schoenhagen P et al. Effect of intensive compared with moderate lipid-lowering therapy on progression of coronary atherosclerosis: a randomized controlled trial. J Am Med Assoc 2004; 291:1132–4.

32. Cannon CP, Braunwald E, McCabe CH et al. Intensive versus moderate lipid lowering with statins after acute coronary syndromes. N Engl J Med 2004; 350:1495–504.
33. LaRosa JC, Grundy SM, Waters DD et al. Intensive lipid lowering with atorvastatin in patients with stable coronary disease. N Engl J Med 2005; 352:1425–35.
34. ALLHAT Officers and Coordinators for the ALLHAT Collaborative Research Group. Major outcomes in moderately hypercholesterolemic, hypertensive patients randomised to pravastatin vs usual care. J Am Med Assoc 2002; 288: 2998–3007.
35. Ridker PM, Cannon CP, Morrow D et al. C-reactive protein levels and outcomes after statin therapy. N Engl J Med 2005; 352:20–8.
36. Nissen SE, Tuzcu EM, Schoenhagen P et al. Statin therapy, LDL cholesterol, C-reactive protein, and coronary artery disease. N Engl J Med 2005; 352:29–38.
37. Goldberg A, Alagona P, Capuzzi DM et al. Multiple-dose efficacy and safety of an extended-release form of niacin in the management of hyperlipidemia. Am J Cardiol 2000; 85:1100–5.
38. Knopp RH, Dujovne CA, Le Beaut et al. Evaluation of the efficacy, safety, and tolerability of ezetimibe in primary hypercholesterolaemia: a pooled analysis from two controlled phase III clinical studies. Int J Clin Prac 2003; 57:363–8.
39. Bucher HC, Hengstler P, Schindler C, Meier G. n-3 polyunsaturated fatty acids in coronary heart disease: a meta-analysis of randomised controlled trials. Am J Med 2002; 112:298–304.
40. Miettinen TA, Strandberg TE, Gylling H, for the Finnish Investigators of the Scandinavian Simvastatin Survival Study Group. Noncholesterol sterols and cholesterol lowering by long-term simvastatin treatment in coronary patients. Arterioscler Thromb Vasc Biol 2000; 20: 1340–6.
41. Davidson MH, McGarry T, Bettis R et al. Ezetimibe coadministered with simvastatin in patients with primary hypercholesterolemia. J Am Coll Cardiol 2002; 40:2125–34.
42. Gagne C, Gaudet D, Bruckert E et al for the Ezetimibe Study Group. Efficacy and safety of ezetimibe coadministered with atorvastatin or simvastatin in patients with homozygous familial hypercholesterolemia. Circulation 2002; 105:2469–75.
43. Catapano A, Brady WE, King TR, Palmisano J. Lipid altering-efficacy of ezetimibe co-administered with simvastatin compared with rosuvastatin: a meta-analysis of pooled data from 14 clinical trials. Curr Med Res Opin 2005; 21:1123–30.
44. Ballantyne CM, Abate N, Yuan Z et al. Dose-comparison study of the combination of ezetimibe and simvastatin (Vytorin) versus atorvastatin in patients with hypercholes-terolaemia: the Vytorin Versus Atorvastatin (VYVA) study. Am Heart J 2005; 149: 464–73.
45. Ballantyne CM, Herd JA, Ferlic LL et al. Influence of low HDL on progression of coronary artery disease and response to fluvastatin therapy. Circulation 1999; 99: 736–43.
46. Brousseau ME, Schaefer EJ, Wolfe ML et al. Effects of an inhibitor of cholesteryl ester transfer protein on HDL cholesterol. N Engl J Med 2004; 350:1505–15.

8

Management issues in primary care

Introduction • Patient assessment • Healthy living • Treatment of individuals at
lower ranges of cardiovascular risk • Initiating statins in primary care • Targets and
how to achieve them • Troubleshooting statin side-effects • Developing structured
care and quality assurance

INTRODUCTION

It is remarkable how the treatment of lipid disorders has moved in just over a
decade from the domain of a few interested secondary care specialists to become a
mainstream activity for all primary care professionals. Clearly, this represents an
appreciation of the burden of atherosclerotic vascular disease at large, the clarifica-
tion of the central, causative role of dyslipidaemia and the emergence of incontro-
vertible evidence of benefit from lipid-modifying trials.

The high prevalence of dyslipidaemia in developed countries means that its
management is largely a primary care problem. In order to optimize patient management in this setting, primary care must identify and treat patients with a high
global cardiovascular risk according to national guidelines, achieve cholesterol and
low density lipoprotein (LDL) cholesterol goals and finally, develop and maintain
pathways of care which ensure target achievement and long-term compliance
within a quality assured system.

PATIENT ASSESSMENT

For secondary prevention in patients with pre-existing atherosclerotic disease –
coronary heart disease (CHD), stroke and transient ischaemic attack (TIA), and
peripheral arterial disease (PAD) – the decision to treat is straightforward. Diabetes
is now accepted as a cardiovascular disease risk equivalent and national guidelines
are unanimous in recommending lipid-lowering treatment for these patients too.

For primary prevention, cardiovascular or CHD risk is calculated using mathematical functions derived from the findings of large databases as described in
Chapters 5 and 6. Treatment thresholds for primary prevention differ between the
major guidelines such that the latest Joint British Recommendations identify a
threshold of >20% / 10 year cardiovascular risk (equivalent to a 10-year CHD risk
of >15%), whereas NCEP ATP III and European recommendations advise
treatment when 10-year CHD risk exceeds 20% or 10-year risk of cardiovascular
death is >5%.[1-3]

Discerning cardiovascular risk status is certainly not intuitive and the risk assessment algorithms and charts, as promoted by the major guidelines, are enormously
helpful in treatment decisions. Many practitioners struggle with the common

Table 8.1   Situations where cardiovascular risk assessment may underestimate risk, with solutions advised by the Joint British Recommendations[1]

Family history of premature CVD <55 years ♂, <65 years ♀	(increase % risk by ×1.3)
Extremes of risk factors (SBP > 160 mmHg or TC : HDL-C > 6)	
Blood pressure and lipid values modified by treatment	(use pre-treatment values)
Ethnic origin	(increase % risk by ×1.4 if from Indian subcontinent)
Impaired glucose tolerance or microalbuminuria	
High triglycerides	
Women with premature menopause	
Age nearing the end of each age category	

SBP, systolic blood pressure; TC, total cholesterol; HDL-C, high density lipoprotein cholesterol.

dyslipidaemia of middle-aged women in whom quite high levels of cholesterol are often seen in conjunction with raised high density lipoprotein (HDL) cholesterol. Placing the total cholesterol to HDL cholesterol ratio in the context of the other risk factors present allows a treatment decision to be made.

Despite the illusion of precision, however, cardiovascular risk assessment is a blunt tool. The accuracy is dependent on the nature of the formative databases themselves, which may over or underestimate risk in different populations. For example, risk is considerably underestimated in certain ethnic populations, such as Indo-Asians. In addition, the risk factor of smoking is treated dichotomously ('smoker'/'non-smoker') discounting the dose-dependent effects of smoking larger amounts. Table 8.1 details a number of situations where risk calculations are potentially unreliable and may underestimate cardiovascular risk.

With these reservations, and the limitations expressed in Chapter 5, it is important to see the current state of cardiovascular risk assessment as a 'tool to guide' rather than 'dictate' practice. Despite this, conventional risk assessment, particularly based on Framingham data, is the best tool we have until such time as an extended range of risk factors or non-invasive clinical testing becomes validated and available.

HEALTHY LIVING

While national guidelines indicate which individuals should or should not be offered drug treatment to reduce their level of cardiovascular risk, it is important to remember to give advice about healthy living to all individuals, irrespective of their defined level of risk or prescribed treatment. The benefits of optimizing weight, eating a healthy diet, increasing physical activity and stopping smoking are clear but, sadly, lifestyle measures are often poorly implemented in practice through lack of expertise, time and conviction.

Optimizing weight

The over-consumption of energy-dense diets, rich in fat and carbohydrate, coupled with reduced physical activity are the reasons behind the growing trend in many societies towards obesity. Losing 5–10% of weight is an achievable target and has been shown to lead to notable reductions in blood pressure and markers of thrombogenic and inflammatory potential as well as improving the lipid profile and insulin sensitivity.[4]

As noted previously, there is a close correlation between waist circumference, visceral obesity and the profile of the metabolic syndrome, such that the rate of obesity related complications is increased in men when waist circumference exceeds a certain limit. Although there is debate about the limit, in men the risk of complications is increased at 94 cm and substantially increased over 102 cm. In women, the values are 80 cm and 88 cm, respectively.[5] Recent studies support the benefits of reducing waist circumference to improve metabolic markers and cardiovascular risk.[6] Waist circumference should be used as an additional measurement to further the assessment of individuals at high cardiovascular risk, and once integrated into primary care practice should assume similar importance to measures of blood pressure and cholesterol.

Eating healthily

The traditional cholesterol-lowering diet is characterized by a low intake of total and saturated fat and dietary cholesterol, with part substitution by mono- and polyunsaturated fats and increased amounts of complex carbohydrates. For both health professionals and patients the recommendations are difficult to conceptualize and few possess the interpretative skills required to incorporate the recommendations into the practicalities of everyday eating. In addition, in 1998, a meta-analysis of 19 randomized controlled trials showed only modest benefits for cholesterol-lowering diets in free-living people.[7] With moderate intensity diets, a disappointing reduction of only 3% in serum cholesterol is seen and only 6% reduction with more rigorous regimes.

Recognition of the need for a more global approach to the dietary prevention of cardiovascular disease than the traditional cholesterol-lowering diet is shown by two key dietary studies, the Lyon Diet Heart Study and the Diet and Reinfarction Trial (DART).[5,6] The Lyon Diet Heart Study tested a Mediterranean-type diet against 'a prudent Western diet' in a CHD secondary prevention setting.[8] After nearly four years, CHD deaths and non-fatal myocardial infarction were significantly reduced by 72%, albeit with wide confidence intervals. The benefits of the study diet lay beyond differences in blood pressure and cholesterol as comparison of the control and experimental groups showed no significant differences between them. A key component of the Mediterranean study diet was α-linolenic acid, an n-3 polyunsaturated fatty acid found in the green tissue of plants. By consuming phytoplankton, fish evolve longer chain n-3 polyunsaturates which in a number of studies have been shown to have cardioprotective properties. In DART, also a secondary prevention trial, the group assigned to eating oily fish twice a week showed a surprisingly high reduction in all cause mortality of 29%.[9]

It is clear that additional nutrients exert lipid-modifying effects and some of these are mentioned in Chapter 3. Of principal importance are the roles of plant (phyto-)sterols, soy protein and complex carbohydrates.

Phytosterols in plants have analogous functions to cholesterol in animals in maintaining cell membrane integrity. Over 50 years of research has demonstrated the ability of phytosterols to reduce cholesterol, and recently the finding that, when esterified, plant sterols and stanols (saturated sterols) become soluble in other fats has led to the commercial development of a range of margarines, spreads and other food vehicles now widely available to the general public. A meta-analysis of 41 trials of the efficacy of sterols and stanols suggests that a mean daily dose of 2 g of either will reduce LDL cholesterol by 10.1% with no significant difference between the two.[10]

In those with higher baseline cholesterol, 25 g of soy protein per day, as part of a diet low in saturated fat and cholesterol, reduces LDL cholesterol by about 6%.[11] Larger reductions are obtained when soy protein is substituted completely for animal protein due to the additional reduction in saturated fat, but there seems to be no effect in individuals with low serum cholesterol.

Dietary patterns rich in complex carbohydrates are associated with decreased risk of cardiovascular disease. Part of the effect results from the actions of insoluble fibre which promotes satiety by slowing gastric emptying and helps to control calorie intake and therefore weight. In addition, certain soluble fibres (such as oat bran and psyllium) have a small LDL cholesterol lowering quality of about 2–3%, which is about the same as substituting unsaturated fats for saturated fats.[12]

Using a 'portfolio' of measures, incorporating plant sterols, soy protein and viscous fibre into an experimental diet, Jenkins has shown a reduction of LDL cholesterol of as much as 29%, equivalent to the effect of a low-dose statin.[13] Clearly, there is more to healthy eating than traditional cholesterol lowering regimes and the guidelines of the American Heart Association are recommended (Table 8.2).[14]

Table 8.2 American Heart Association dietary guidelines for the prevention of cardiovascular disease[14]

1. **Use foods and dietary patterns with broad health benefits**
   Fruit and vegetables five times a day
   Increased grain products (especially wholegrain cereals) six times a day
   Fat-free and low-fat dairy products
   Fish twice a week
   Legumes, poultry and lean meat

2. **Place greater emphasis on weight loss and obesity control**
   Match intake of energy to needs to prevent obesity and maintain a healthy body weight
   Limit intake of foods with high caloric value (especially sugars)
   Achieve a level of appropriate physical activity for weight maintenance or loss

3. **Maintain a desirable blood cholesterol, lipoprotein profile and blood pressure**
   Limit intake of saturated fatty acids (<10%) and cholesterol (<300 mg/day)
   Minimize trans fats
   Substitute with grains and unsaturated fatty acids (especially from vegetables, fish, legumes and nuts)
   Limit salt to <6 g/day
   Limit alcohol to two drinks per day for men, one for women
   Maintain healthy body weight
   Emphasize fruit and vegetables and low fat products

4. **Target special populations and higher risk subgroups with individual approaches**
   Older individuals, children, those with elevated LDL cholesterol, pre-existing cardiovascular disease, diabetes mellitus, congestive heart failure or kidney disease

Exercising regularly

A number of studies have shown that repeated, moderate amounts of aerobic activity result in reductions in total cholesterol, LDL cholesterol and triglycerides and elevations in HDL cholesterol. Plasma triglycerides show the greatest improvement, which relates to increased activity of lipoprotein lipase in muscles and adipose tissue. The changes correlate with the degree of fitness achieved and the intensity of the activity, such that very high levels of activity can reduce LDL cholesterol by as much as 1 mmol/L and raise HDL cholesterol significantly. For most sedentary individuals, the current recommendation advising 30 minutes of moderate intensity physical activity on most days seems a sensible starting point, but more exercise will confer greater benefit.

TREATMENT OF INDIVIDUALS AT LOWER RANGES OF CARDIOVASCULAR RISK

Treating dyslipidaemia at the levels of cardiovascular risk endorsed by national and international guidelines is an enormous task and in the UK nearly five million people under 70 qualify for treatment with a statin. The evidence base, however, shows that healthy eating and the use of statins are effective, even in populations at levels of cardiovascular risk lower than the guideline thresholds. AFCAPS/ TEXCAPS showed that using a statin and a low fat dietary approach in a primary prevention population, whose 10-year risk of CHD was just 6%, was effective (albeit with lower absolute benefit).[15] It must be remembered that treatment thresholds reflect not only the evidence base for benefit, but also the absolute amount of benefit derived, the practicality of dealing with the numbers of people involved and the affordability of drug and infrastructure costs. With this in mind in 2004, amid worldwide scrutiny, the UK government sanctioned the availability of simvastatin 10 mg 'over the counter' (OTC) under pharmacist supervision. Making statins available OTC means that individuals at 'medium' risk, who are just below the intervention threshold (i.e. 10–20% / 10 year cardiovascular event risk, the orange band of the Joint British Societies guidelines[1]), can benefit from cardiovascular risk reduction if they so choose and at their own expense.

Risk assessment is simplified for pharmacists and OTC statin can be offered to:

- Men over 55 years;
- Men aged 45–55 years or women over 55, who have a family history of CHD, who smoke, are overweight or of South Asian origin. Higher-risk individuals are referred for treatment to their doctors.

The uptake of OTC statins has been slow and probably reflects the relative complexity of the risk-based approach. In addition there have been a number of professional concerns, chiefly reflecting the ability of pharmacists to manage the programme (especially in the longer term), worries about inappropriate use, side-effects, social inequities and upstream effects on workload in primary care. Another concern has been the lack of any obligation that serum cholesterol should be measured before OTC simvastatin is dispensed.

INITIATING STATINS IN PRIMARY CARE

Although their efficacy varies, statins are all highly effective in reducing total cholesterol and LDL cholesterol and are the mainstay of the treatment for dyslipidaemia. The initiation of a statin for dyslipidaemia is the final step in the pathway leading from the discovery of dyslipidaemia itself, through cardiovascular risk assessment and ultimately to the decision to prescribe, based on the risks and benefits pertinent to the individual concerned.

We have seen in Chapter 4 that measuring the lipoprotein profile on two occasions increases the accuracy of assessment and that at least one measurement should be fasting. An important feature of the assessment of abnormal lipid levels is to exclude the causes of secondary hyperlipidaemia. Commonly these include obesity, diabetes, hypothyroidism and excessive alcohol intake but a more extensive list is covered in Chapter 1. Fasting blood glucose, liver and renal function tests and measurement of thyroid stimulating hormone are useful investigations before initiating treatment.

Even if the patient's level of cardiovascular risk mandates treatment, the practitioner still has some decisions to make before prescribing. Considerations include age, prognosis, the presence of concomitant disease, the possibility of drug interactions and the likelihood of compliance. Statins should not be given to young children, except in the rare situation of familial hypercholesterolaemia with a bad family history, and they are also unsuitable for pregnant or lactating women. Although the absolute risk of cardiovascular disease is higher in older patients and the benefits of statins may be significant, statins take time to improve outcome and the older patient needs to have a reasonable life expectancy in order to benefit. Particular consideration needs to be given to concomitant renal and hepatic disease, the exclusion of hypothyroidism and other pharmacotherapy.

By and large, statins are remarkably well tolerated and it is important to pass this information on to the patient. Over 100 million people worldwide now take statins. Although the chances of acute myositis and rhabdomyolysis are rare (about once per 50 000 patient-years of treatment) it is also important to indicate this possibility, together with an action plan to seek prompt help. The symptoms felt by the patient are usually of a generalized muscle discomfort and weakness akin to the myalgia of the first days of 'flu.

The effect of treatment can be assessed by follow-up blood testing after 4 weeks, and encouraging the patient's interest in the results is a useful strategy for fostering patient compliance. It is also reasonable to check the liver enzyme alanine transferase (ALT) at the time of the first post-treatment check.

TARGETS AND HOW TO ACHIEVE THEM

Most health care professionals now work to target values in the treatment of dyslipidaemia for the reduction of cardiovascular risk. Different guidelines identify different target values for total and LDL cholesterol and desirable levels for HDL cholesterol, non-HDL cholesterol and triglycerides and these are outlined in Chapter 6. It should be borne in mind that the targets are derived by consensus panels and have little evidence from clinical outcome trials per se. Many patients in the clinical trials failed to achieve target levels, yet, presumably, derived benefit from treatment. Prescribers must, therefore, weigh up the benefit from the specific settings of randomized trials with the extrapolated benefit derived from the relative surrogate of achieving target lipid values.

In addition to achieving lipid targets, other measures to reduce cardiovascular risk must not be forgotten. In particular, a healthy lifestyle, measures to ensure blood pressure and glycaemic control and the use of guardian drugs such as antiplatelet agents, β-blockers and angiotensin converting inhibitors or angiotensin receptor blockers where appropriate.

Patient compliance

Poor compliance is clearly one of the factors responsible for the 'implementation gap' between the potential benefits indicated by the evidence base and actual clinical practice. The true extent of non-compliance or non-persistence with prescribed lipid-lowering therapy is unknown, but small surveys suggest that after one year barely 50% of patients continue with their medication, a finding in line with the experience of other long-term treatments, such as anti-hypertensive drugs. Technically, a distinction should be made between full non-compliance and partial compliance. Partial compliance is invariably the rule and overall, patients take only three-quarters of medication prescribed.

Compliance is known to improve both before and after an encounter with a health professional. This emphasizes the potential of ongoing support by an interested health professional with their patient. Helpful tactics for enhancing compliance are shown in Table 8.3 and also listed by the American National Cholesterol Education Program.[16]

Strategies for achieving target lipid levels

Having ensured that the patient is compliant with both lifestyle and pharmacological interventions, a number of strategies exist to ensure lipid target success.

1. *Statin dose titration*. This has been the traditional approach but is often ignored as patients tend to stay on low, starter doses of drugs which, for a number of reasons, fail to be titrated upwards.
2. *'Right first time'* – using a drug that is efficacious enough to get most patients to target at the chosen starter dose. This is more time efficient and may be more agreeable to both doctors and patients.

Table 8.3 Tactics for enhancing compliance with lipid-lowering treatment

1. Teach the patient about the treatment regime – instructions should be simple but comprehensive.
2. Help the patient to remember to take the medication – tailor doses to daily habits.
3. Reinforce compliance – ask about it, chart lipid responses, provide encouragement.
4. Anticipate common problems and teach the patient how to manage them.
5. Involve a family member or friend in the patient's therapy programme.
6. Establish a supportive relationship with the patient – provide ongoing updates and information about the patient's illness and treatment.
7. Provide individualized services for patients who avoid compliance.
8. Assess barriers.
   - Physical   e.g. poor vision, forgetfulness
   - Access   e.g. transportation, income and time
   - Attitude   e.g. fatalism
   - Therapy   e.g. complexity and real or perceived side effects
   - Social   e.g. family instability
   - Faulty perceptions e.g. denial

3. *Switching* – if an inadequate response is found with one drug, then switch to a more effective one.
4. *Combination therapy* – adding a second drug with a different mechanism of action to produce a complementary response. Most combinations involve a statin with a fibrate, ezetimibe or a resin, fish oil or nicotinic acid.
5. *Referral to a lipid clinic*. This may be appropriate for patients who fail to show an effective response to treatment, those with extreme values or familial dyslipidaemia and those special cases requiring more extensive investigations. Such may include apolipoprotein analysis, enzyme testing or DNA genotyping, or the help of paediatric, cardiology, nephrology, neurology, vascular surgery and HIV specialists.

TROUBLESHOOTING STATIN SIDE-EFFECTS

In the many double-blind, randomized, placebo-controlled trials of statins the side-effect rates have been very low, without significant differences in adverse-event withdrawal between study groups. In clinical practice, occasional patients are unable to tolerate statins because of mild (usually upper) gastrointestinal side-effects, but the main side-effect encountered (and much feared by practitioners) is myopathy. Despite its importance, myopathy is rare and exact reasons for its occurrence are not fully understood. It is more common in those with concomitant illness, in women, those of small body mass and the elderly.

Myopathy is associated with a rise in the muscle enzyme, creatinine (phospho)kinase (CPK or CK). A CK rise of greater than ten times the upper limit of normal is seen in acute myositis, and if this continues without drug withdrawal severe muscle breakdown (rhabdomyolysis) can occur, leading to acute renal failure and potentially death. CK levels vary enormously, even in individuals not on treatment, and can rise markedly with muscle injury or energetic activity. For this reason random CK checks are unhelpful and should only be performed in symptomatic patients, when myopathy is suspected. CK elevations up to five or even ten times normal can be acceptable in asymptomatic patients.

Some patients experience myalgia without CK rise and this can bear a close temporal relationship to their statin. Other statins, lower doses or combination therapy with ezetimibe may allow the patient to continue with lipid-lowering medication. Anecdotally, coenzyme Q10 reportedly helps some patients but more research is needed to confirm this.

High plasma levels of statins are myotoxic, and drug interactions which raise statin levels are an important cause of myopathy. Statins are mostly metabolized by the P450 isoenzyme system in the liver, a pathway common to the metabolism of a number of other drugs which therefore show the potential for interaction (Table 8.4).

Of the statins, simvastatin, atorvastatin, lovastatin and cerivastatin are metabolized through the 3A4 isoenzyme and have more potential to interact with drugs like erythromycin and ciclosporine. The interaction between cerivastatin and the partly 3A4 metabolized fibrate, gemfibrozil, was partly responsible for its withdrawal in 2001. In this category, grapefruit juice, even in small quantities can increase statin levels by the action of 6',7'-dihydroxybergamottin on 3A4 metabolism.[18] Grapefruit juice is therefore 'off-the-menu' for patients taking 3A4 metabolized statins. Statins can be suspended for short courses of macrolide therapy

Table 8.4 The metabolism of various drugs through the human cytochrome P450 isoenzyme system. (After Ballantyne et al[17])

CYP3A4	CYP2D6	CYP2C19	CYP2C9
Amiodarone	Amitriptyline	Diazepam	Alprenolol
Amlodipine	Bufaralol	Ibuprofen	Diclofenac
Atorvastatin	Codeine	Mephenytoin	Fluvastatin
Cerivastatin	Debrisoquine	Methylphenobarbital	Pravastatin
Clarithromycin	Dextromethorphan	Omeprazol	Hexobarbital
Cyclosporine A	Encainide	Proguanyl	N-desmethyl-
Diltiazem	Flecainide	Phenytoin	diazepam
Erythromycin	Imipramine		Tolbutamide
Ketoconazole	Metoprolol		Warfarin
Itraconazole	Mibefradil		
Lovastatin	Nortriptyline		
Mibefradil	Perhexiline		
Midazolam	Perphenazine		
Nefazodone	Propafenone		
Nifedipine	Propranolol		
Protease inhibitors	Sparteine		
Quinidine	Thioridazine		
Sildenafil	Timolol		
Simvastatin			
Terbinafine			

Rosuvastatin has 10% metabolism through CYP2C9 and CYP2C19]

but for chronic treatments such as ciclosporine, non-3A4 metabolized statins should be chosen. Fluvastatin and pravastatin are metabolized through CYP2C9 and have fewer potential interactions (fluvastatin has been used in a major clinical trial with ciclosporine). Rosuvastatin is excreted mostly unchanged with only 10% metabolized through 2C9 and 2C19, but ciclosporin still raises rosuvastatin levels several-fold.

Clearly, despite their shared mode of action, all statins are not the same. Additional differences exist in their efficacy and various pharmacological properties such as half-life and lipophilicity. For example, the half-lives of atorvastatin and rosuvastatin are long, meaning that they can be taken at any time of day, whereas the other statins with shorter half-lives should be taken at night. The differences between statins are such that where one is not tolerated it is well worth trying an alternative.

Liver enzymes can also rise occasionally with statin therapy, although this is rarely important in the absence of underlying liver disease, and in asymptomatic individuals a rise in alanine transaminase (ALT) of up to three times normal is acceptable. Statin therapy is conventionally stopped if ALT exceeds three times normal on two separate occasions, but some experts are beginning to debate this, feeling that the positive cardiovascular outcomes of statin therapy outweigh any consequences of mild liver enzyme changes. If liver enzymes are abnormal prior to statin initiation, then the cause of the abnormality should be defined. A common difficulty is seen with patients with metabolic syndrome, where fatty infiltration of the liver (seen as an echo-bright ultrasound) is often associated with mild liver enzyme disturbance. Hepatitis, alcohol excess, other drugs and rarely haemochromatosis and α-1-antitrypsin deficiency are important causes of ALT abnormality, often accompanied by an elevated γ-glutamyl transferase.

DEVELOPING STRUCTURED CARE AND QUALITY ASSURANCE

The existence of the implementation gap between expectation and reality underlines the failure, in many practices, to develop systematic care pathways for patients needing cardiovascular disease prevention interventions. The computer is central to the efforts of most successful practices, and appropriate coding, database construction, the use of templates and call and recall systems, all enhance the delivery of care. Much research has focused on the role of the primary care nurse, and data from the Grampian region in Scotland show significant improvements in the level of interventions and even the death rate, at 4.7 years, in CHD patients attending nurse-led clinics.[19]

Nurses already have established roles in chronic disease management in asthma and diabetes in primary care. As the aims are so similar, a logical step would be to expand practice diabetes clinics to become cardiovascular disease prevention clinics. Primary care organizations should co-ordinate local activities and facilitate integration with secondary care services. In addition, the role of intermediate care 'specialists' in general practice is likely to expand.

The importance and ease of clinical audit of cholesterol measurements has made them ideal quality indicators. In the UK, GPs are financially rewarded for their performance against a number of clinical audit criteria demonstrating the quality of their care across different fields of clinical practice.[20] For example, in the secondary prevention of CHD, seven quality points are available for ensuring that 90% of CHD patients have a cholesterol recording over the preceding 15 months, and 19 quality points are available if 60% achieve the total cholesterol target of 5.0 mmol/L or below over the same time period. The same standards and time-frames apply to cerebrovascular disease and diabetes, with two and three points available, respectively, for measurement, and five and six points, respectively, for target achievement. Primary health care professionals have had to develop appropriately structured care to facilitate easy recording of data, with built-in audits to anticipate that quality standards will be met. Point accumulation translates into direct performance-pay for the practices, and as a result major improvements in the quality of care have been seen after the scheme's first year.

REFERENCES

1. British Cardiac Society, British Hypertension Society, Diabetes UK, HEART UK, Primary Care Cardiovascular Society, The Stroke Association. JBS2: Joint British Societies' guidelines on prevention of cardiovascular disease in clinical practice. Heart 2005; 91(Suppl V): v1–v52.
2. Third Report of the National Cholesterol Education Program (NCEP) Expert Panel on Detection, Evaluation and Treatment of High Blood Cholesterol in Adults (Adult Treatment Panel III). J Am Med Assoc 2001; 285:2486–97.
3. De Backer G, Ambrosioni E, Borch-Johnsen K et al. European guidelines on cardiovascular disease prevention in clinical practice: Third Joint Task Force of European and other societies on Cardiovascular Disease Prevention in Clinical Practice. Eur Heart J 2003; 24:1601–10.

4. Sharma AM. Adipose tissue: a mediator of cardiovascular risk. Int J Obesity 2002; 26(Suppl4):S5–S7.
5. Lean MEJ, Han TS, Morrison CE. Waist circumference indicates the need for weight management. Br Med J 1995; 311:158–61.
6. Wang Y, Rimm EB, Stampfer MJ et al. Comparison of abdominal adiposity and overall obesity in predicting risk of type 2 diabetes among men. Am J Clin Nutr 2005; 81:555–63.
7. Tang JL, Armitage JM, Lancaster T et al. Systematic review of dietary intervention trials to lower blood cholesterol in free-living subjects. Br Med J 1998; 316:1213–20.
8. De Lorgeril M, Salen P, Martin JL et al. Mediterranean diet, traditional risk factors and the rate of cardiovascular complications after myocardial infarction: the final report of the Lyon Diet Heart Study. Circulation 1999 99:779–85.
9. Burr ML, Fehily AM, Gilbert JF et al. Effects of changes in fat, fish and fiber intakes on Death and Myocardial Reinfarction Trial (DART). Lancet 1989; 2:757–61.
10. Katan MB, Grundy SM, Jones P et al. Efficacy and safety of plant stanols and sterols in the management of blood cholesterol levels. Mayo Clin Proc 2003; 78:965–78.
11. Erdman JW. Soy protein and cardiovascular disease. Circulation 2000; 102:2555–9.
12. Brown L, Rosner B, Willett W et al. Cholesterol-lowering effects of dietary fiber: a meta-analysis. Am J Clin Nutr 1999; 69:30–42.
13. Jenkins DJA, Kendall CWC, Faulkner D et al. A dietary portfolio approach to cholesterol reduction: combined effects of plant sterols, vegetable proteins, and viscous fibers in hypercholesterolaemia. Metab Clin Exp 2002; 51:1596–604.
14. American Heart Association. AHA dietary guidelines: revision. Circulation 2000; 102:2284–99.
15. Down JR, Clearfield M, Weis S et al for the AFCAPS/TexCAPS Research Group. Primary prevention of acute coronary events with lovastatin in men and women with average cholesterol levels: results of AFCAPS/TexCAPS. J Am Med Assoc 1998; 279:1615–22.
16. Expert panel on detection, evaluation and treatment of high blood cholesterol in adults. Executive summary of the third report of the National Cholesterol Education Program (NCEP) expert panel on detection, evaluation and treatment of high blood cholesterol in adults (Adult Treatment Panel III). J Am Med Assoc 2001; 285:2486–97.
17. Ballantyne CM, Corsini A, Davidson MH et al. Risk for myopathy with statin therapy for high-risk patients: expert panel review. Arch Intern Med 2003; 163:553–64.
18. Lilja JJ, Neuvonen M, Neuvonen PJ. Effects of regular consumption of grapefruit juice on the pharmacokinetics of simvastatin. Br J Clin Pharmacol 2004; 58:56–60.
19. Murchie P, Campbell NC, Ritchie LD et al. Secondary prevention clinics for coronary heart disease: four year follow up of a randomised controlled trial in primary care. Br Med J 2003; 326:84–7.
20. British Medical Association and NHS Confederation. Investing in general practice: the new general medical services contract. London: Department of Health, 2003.

Index

Printed and bound by CPI Group (UK) Ltd, Croydon, CR0 4YY

27/10/2024

01779947-0002